UNDERSTANDING MICROINFLAMMATION

THE COMMON LINK BETWEEN AGING, CANCER AND CORONARY DISEASE

KENNETH B. JOHNSON, MD MBA FACC
RAJIV S. DAHIYA, MD

D1400644

ISBN: 1482735385

ISBN 13: 9781482735383

Library of Congress Control Number: 2013904814

CreateSpace Independent Publishing Platform

North Charleston, South Carolina

CONTENTS

FOREWORD

As practitioners of traditional allopathic medicine, we fully understand the utility as well as limitations of current medical practice. When we began our careers in cardiology and oncology, we dedicated our lives to the treatment of two of the most lethal diseases in the world. Our specialties have witnessed some of the greatest progress in medical history, with research in recent decades providing us with remarkable advances in diagnostic modalities as well as pharmacological and procedural treatments for cancer and cardiac disease.

Yet many traditionally trained physicians have their shortcomings in one particular arena—disease prevention. Our discipline was born out of the need to treat diseases once signs and symptoms developed, and that mind-set has remained within the medical profession since time immemorial. Preventing disease has largely been a secondary goal of physicians, although recent paradigm shifts have attempted to incorporate primary prevention and health-care maintenance into most of the major disciplines. Yet it is clear that we, as a whole, have not readily embraced the concepts of prevention, and certainly have not fully exploited the available and abundant science that is at our fingertips.

Without attempting to make excuses for our shortcomings in disease prevention, we do recognize many reasons for physician reluctance in adopting preventive strategies. Principally, we are practitioners of tradition. Even though technology brings us new opportunities almost daily, we are slow to adopt change because it is hard for us to break our time-honored roots in the medical sciences. We often require multiple lines of evidence demonstrating the same effect for us to truly consider changes in our clinical practice. Our actions often hinge on the results of landmark clinical trials, and anything less is viewed with little regard. At times, this perspective can be productive and prevents us from prematurely adopting practices that are not wholly evidence based. At other times, as in the case of preventive medicine, our traditional biases are a hindrance.

Secondly, we often overlook simple therapies and de-emphasize the relevance of modalities such as dietary modification, exercise, and use of vitamins, minerals and other supplements. Although we generally try to get our patients to eat right and exercise, we don't go to extraordinary efforts to educate them in these arenas. Further, we prefer to recommend prescription medicines over supplements, as we are more comfortable in this realm because of our familiarity with pharmacology and our lack of knowledge in herbal or other supplements collectively known as nutraceuticals. Again, the fundamental basis for our behavior here is a bias of tradition.

So this book represents our determination to overcome our traditional boundaries and integrate our in-depth understanding of clinical medicine with new insights into the cellular, molecular, and genetic bases of aging and disease. This integration allows us to gaze beyond our conventional approaches to treating illness and actually create a recipe for disease prevention. With a multimodality approach to primary prevention that incorporates pharmacology, natural supplements, dietary modification, genetic and other laboratory testing we believe that diseases can at least be delayed, and in many cases prevented, at the cellular level. Obviously, no one can live forever, but we hope to present a foundation that will allow us all to live longer, disease-free lives.

Kenneth B. Johnson, MD MBA FACC
Rajiv S. Dahiya, MD

CHAPTER 1:
THE HARSH REALITY

Each year, there are nearly 2.5 million registered deaths in the United States alone. Among these, nearly half are attributable to cardiac disease and cancer, making them the number one and number two killers of Americans, respectively (see table 1). More provocatively, these two diseases claim the lives of more individuals in this country than the next thirteen causes of death combined and contribute to the death of two Americans every sixty seconds! Looking at mortality statistics globally, heart disease retains its number one spot, being the principal cause of death worldwide, and cancer, although not as prominent a killer throughout the world, still falls within the top ten (see table 1). Although medical advancements in procedures, pharmaceuticals, and other therapies have allowed individuals with cardiac disease and cancer to survive and live longer, these two conditions still pose a formidable threat to individuals throughout the world. More critically, traditional medicine has largely focused on disease treatment, and only in recent decades has there been an explosion in research into preventive therapies for these and other ailments.

Perhaps one of the most astonishing revelations in the past decade is that many of the risk factors—identifiable conditions, behaviors, or exposures that increase an individual's chance of contracting a disease—that contribute to the development of cancer and cardiac disease are actually linked, and, more importantly, largely preventable. Traditional disease risk factors are stratified into modifiable and nonmodifiable causes. As the name

1

implies, nonmodifiable risk factors are those over which we have no control, and in the case of coronary disease and cancer, these include gender, family history, and age.

On the other hand, there are myriad conditions that predispose to the development or progression of certain diseases that we can modify through either behavioral changes, medical therapy, nutritional supplementation, or a combination of all of these. In the case of coronary artery disease, modifiable risk factors include tobacco abuse, obesity, inactivity, high cholesterol, high blood pressure, diabetes mellitus, and poor eating habits. Similarly, factors that increase cancer risk include tobacco use, obesity, inactivity, alcohol consumption, radiation exposure, hormone replacement therapy, and exposure to carcinogens (environmental or chemical agents that promote cancer development).

Although many of the cardiac and cancer risks are divergent, there is clear overlap in tobacco abuse, obesity, inactivity, and poor eating habits. Further, as we shall illustrate, recent research has elucidated the fundamental cellular basis behind many of these risk factors, and the mechanisms by which they produce diseases such as coronary atherosclerosis and cancer is through oxidative stress and newly discovered inflammatory pathways. We will reveal that the fundamental link between aging, cancer, and coronary disease development and progression is a complex interaction between a chronic, low-grade state of cellular inflammation known as microinflammation, metainflammation, or parainflammation, as well as destructive oxidative processes. This powerful revelation has led to a critical change in our ability to understand the molecular foundations of not only diseases, but the aging process, or senescence, itself. Appreciating this presents new opportunity and insight into preventing disease and retarding the aging process, rather than simply treating conditions after the fact. By recognizing the interactions between molecular and cellular physiology and traditional risk factors, we can approach risks in a multidimensional fashion, attenuate or eliminate them, and reduce our chances of capitulating to the two primary modes of death in this country.

RANK	LEADING CAUSES OF DEATH IN THE UNITED STATES AND WORLD	
	CAUSE OF DEATH IN US	CAUSE OF DEATH IN THE WORLD
1	Heart Disease	Heart Disease
2	Cancer	Stroke and other Cerebrovascular Disease
3	Chronic Lung Disease	Lower Respiratory Infections
4	Cerebrovascular Disease	Chronic Lung Disease
5	Accidents (Unintentional Injuries)	Diarrheal Diseases
6	Alzheimer's Disease	HIV/AIDS
7	Diabetes Mellitus	Trachea, Bronchus, Lung Cancers
8	Influenza and Pneumonia	Tuberculosis
9	Nephritis, Nephritic Syndrome, and Nephrosis	Diabetes Mellitus
10	Intentional Self-Harm (Suicide)	Road Traffic Accidents

Table 1: Top 10 Causes of Death in the United States and Worldwide
Adapted from Centers for Disease Control Vital Statistics and the World Health Organization Global Health Observatory Data Repository[1,2]

CHAPTER 2:
UNDERSTANDING OXIDATIVE STRESS

Oxidative stress describes a physiological condition in our bodies that results from a disruption in the balance between harmful and nonharmful products created from the oxygen that we metabolize to fuel our cellular functions. Oxygen is obviously essential to life, but when disruptions in cellular processes occur because of disease states or other physical stress, it can be used to form toxic substances within our bodies. The harmful byproducts of oxygen metabolism are generally termed "oxidants," whereas the beneficial derivatives are denoted as "antioxidants," and their balance is critical to maintain appropriate cellular function. The equilibrium between oxidants and antioxidants is known as our redox state, and under conditions where the balance is shifted toward excess oxidants, we are said to be under oxidative stress.

There are two principal sources of oxidants within us—mitochondria (see figure 1) and phagocytes. Mitochondria are self-contained factories within our cells that are responsible for producing units of energy in the form of a molecule called adenosine triphosphate (ATP). ATP is considered the energy currency for all cells within the body and is utilized to fuel most bodily processes, including muscle contraction, protein synthesis, transport of substances in and out of cells, and myriad other activities.

Phagocytes are a family of cells that possess the ability to attack and engulf other cells or circulating debris and principally function within our immune systems. Phagocytes can be viewed as ravenous scavengers that travel through our bloodstream and tissues, devouring substances that are usually harmful to us in some way. Some phagocytes possess mitochondria of their own (one example is the macrophage) and can produce oxidants much the same way as other cells with normally functioning mitochondria do. Other phagocytes lack mitochondria (one example is the neutrophil), but possess the ability to induce chemical reactions that ultimately result in oxidants that can be used as weapons for our immune systems.

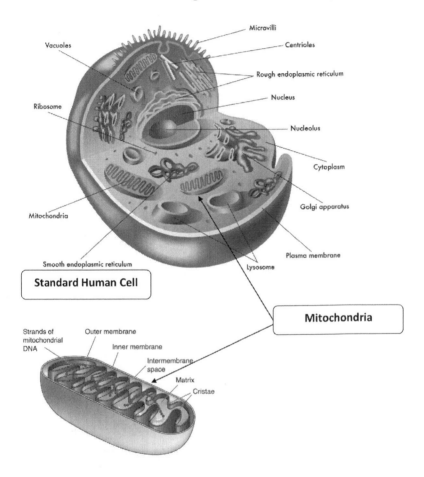

Figure 1: Mitochondria A standard human cell is depicted with multiple energy-producing mitochondria. Cells may contain a variable amount of these energy factories depending on their specific function.

In any case, a key step in the activity of either mitochondria or phagocytes is to utilize oxygen in specific chemical reactions. In some cases, an oxygen molecule will be transformed, either intentionally or unintentionally, into an oxidant byproduct known as a reactive oxygen species (ROS).

Reactive oxygen species are so named because of their relatively unstable nature, which increases their propensity to participate in chemical reactions (both desired and undesired). ROS are generally stratified into two categories: free radicals or nonradicals. Free radicals are atoms or molecules that possess an imbalance of charges such that one or more of the electrons in the atom or molecule is unpaired. Typical examples of this include the superoxide radical, which is an oxygen molecule with an extra electron (designated as O_2-) or the hydroxyl ion (designated OH-). Nonradical ROS are still highly reactive, but do not possess an imbalance of electrons and include molecules such as hydrogen peroxide (H_2O_2) and nitric oxide (NO).

Under normal conditions, approximately 1%–5% of the oxygen utilized within human mitochondrial cells is converted to reactive oxygen species. As a result, they are considered a normal byproduct in low concentrations and even serve some beneficial functions within the body at these sparse levels. Superoxide, for example, is produced as a toxic weapon that can help destroy invading microorganisms. Similarly, hydrogen peroxide, which is more stable than superoxide, is involved in a process known as redox signaling, which allows different cells to interpret information about and respond to stimuli within their environment. Such biological signaling is paramount to the activation of key enzyme systems and even the stimulation of deoxyribonucleic acid (DNA) synthesis.[1-3]

Under pathological conditions and physiological stress, ROS can be produced in excess and liberated from the mitochondria or its parent cell and have the potential to induce oxidant-related damage both to the cell that produced it and to other surrounding ones. Understanding these processes, a revised definition of oxidative stress is an imbalance in the redox state of our cells or tissues resulting in a concentration of reactive oxygen species that exceeds our cell's antioxidant capacity.

Although oxidative stress has been understood for decades, and antioxidant therapy has been advocated in the healthy living literature by nutritional experts and in nutritional supplement stores, the concept of treating redox imbalance has largely been ignored by the medical community and the public at large. Perhaps there are many reasons for this, but among them is likely the fact that treating oxidative stress doesn't tend to produce readily observable effects or noticeable changes in the way we feel. Whereas antibiotics make people feel better by killing bacteria that cause us to have symptoms such as fever or cough, and pain medicines attenuate or alleviate the pain of arthritis or injury, antioxidants generally do not induce any perceptible effects. Thus, redox imbalance becomes a silent killer and goes largely untreated.

Yet there are other silent killers in medicine that still receive treatment. High blood pressure, for example, is principally diagnosed in asymptomatic individuals, after which medical practitioners usually prescribe medicines to lower the blood pressure. Although some patients with extremely high blood pressure complain of symptoms such as headache, chest pain, difficulty breathing, or visual disturbances, the majority have no symptoms whatsoever. As a result, when patients are treated for high blood pressure, they most often experience no observable effect, or, in many cases, actually feel worse because they develop side effects from the medicines. Nonetheless, as practitioners of medicine, we understand the importance of long-term blood pressure control to reduce the risks of stroke and heart attack, and advocate lifelong use of antihypertensive agents.

So why don't we approach oxidative stress in the same manner? Again, there probably isn't a simple answer to this, but it likely relates to two fundamental truths: (1) the data on antioxidant efficacy is not nearly as robust as the data on high blood pressure control, and (2) as we previously iterated, traditionally trained health-care providers are largely reluctant to embrace change and nontraditional therapies. There is no argument about the breadth of data available on antioxidants, but, as we shall see, there is plenty of evidence to support their use in different settings. Moreover, when reacting as a traditional practitioner and performing a cost-benefit analysis on most antioxidants, it is obvious that the relative cost or downside is minimal compared to many prescription and nonprescription medicines. As we move forward in our attempts to conquer disease and aging, we must consider the evidence for preventive therapies in this light and embrace new concepts and strategies that can potentially prevent harmful physiological processes.

As new, provocative insights into the molecular basis of aging and disease emerge, and microinflammation and its interaction with oxidative stress has entered the arena as a formidable threat, now, more than ever, we must embrace a nontraditional view for disease prevention. By no means does this involve ignoring traditional science. Rather, it means approaching prevention with a more open mind and considering other options that show promise in the scientific literature as long as their cost-benefit ratio favors a net advantageous effect. Attacking oxidative pathways where they originate and inhibiting the interface between oxidative stress and microinflammation is paramount to any primary prevention strategy.

OXIDATIVE CELL DAMAGE

As described previously, ROS are normal byproducts of cellular metabolism, and we are usually insulated from their damaging effects by a sophisticated antioxidant system. Moreover, in lower concentrations, the oxidants produced by our cells can serve useful functions. Higher levels of ROS resulting in redox imbalance can occur, however, and contribute to a host of untoward effects. Redox disparity generally occurs in three fundamental ways: (1) Our standard processes, under stress conditions, can produce an excess of oxidant substances by way of our normal cellular machinery. (2) Oxidative overload can be the result of decreased cellular antioxidant capacity, which can occur via decreased gene-encoded production of or reduced dietary uptake of vital antioxidants. (3) Many other substances, including drugs, hormones, and other chemical agents, have clearly been shown, either directly or indirectly, to instigate the production of ROS.[1-3] By whatever mechanism, when oxidative stress ensues, metabolic derangements and cellular damage can produce a multitude of deleterious effects on our bodies.

Examining superoxide again, it is established that excess amounts of this species can escape the mitochondria and readily interact with an enzyme system known as superoxide dismutase, which can rapidly convert the superoxide into hydrogen peroxide and free oxygen. This hydrogen peroxide is essentially the same agent that can be purchased in a grocery store and is used for cleaning, bleaching, or even as a propellant in liquid rocket engines. By picturing how hydrogen peroxide foams when in contact with blood, it is not difficult to imagine how corrosive it could be to cells or tissues within us!

As noted previously, hydrogen peroxide is a nonradical ROS and is considered a powerful oxidizing agent or oxidant (meaning that it readily accepts electrons in chemical reactions). Under normal conditions, the small quantities of hydrogen peroxide that are produced function positively in the cellular signaling pathway describe previously. Its concentration is normally kept in check by enzymes known as peroxidases that are responsible for converting it to water and oxygen. If the amount of hydrogen peroxide produced, however, exceeds the available supply of peroxidase, it becomes a potent circulating toxin that can damage DNA or RNA, impair lipid and protein function, and inactivate certain enzyme systems.

Lipids, or fat, certain proteins, and DNA are cellular constituents that are among the most sensitive to oxidative damage. A specific configuration of lipids, known as fatty acids, form the backbone of all cellular membranes and possess important functions in maintaining the integrity of the cell itself. Like a security wall surrounding a castle, the fatty acid–rich membrane is responsible for keeping desirable constituents within the cell and preventing undesirable agents from entering it. Incorporated within the fatty acids are proteins, which function as gates that control the entry and exit of ions, nutrients, and other substances. Oxidative damage to the membrane itself or these transport proteins can lead to derangement in the influx or efflux of important substances, contributing ultimately to cellular dysfunction.[4]

In addition to transport proteins involved in cell membrane stability, other proteins known as transcription factors can readily be affected by oxidative stress.[5] As the name implies, these small molecules are responsible for regulating the process of gene transcription (see figure 2).

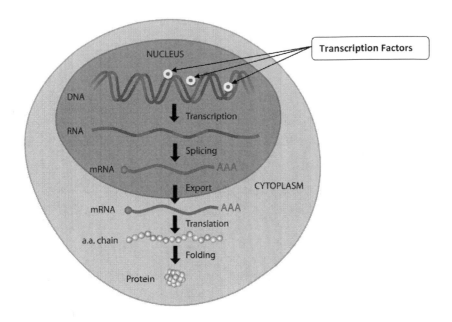

Figure 2: Gene Expression The original DNA molecule that resides in the nucleus of a cell first undergoes transcription, during which a complementary RNA strand is created from the DNA template. Transcription factors attach to the DNA molecule and either promote or inhibit transcription of certain information from that region of the DNA molecule. The RNA strand undergoes some modifications to become what is known as messenger RNA (mRNA), which is then transported out of the nucleus, into the cytoplasm. Translation occurs next, where amino acid building blocks are made from the specific pattern encoded by the mRNA molecule. The amino acid chain then folds into a predetermined configuration to create the specific protein encoded by the original DNA molecule.

This is the first step in gene expression, during which DNA is used as a template to create a complementary RNA strand, which then ultimately can be translated into a functioning protein. By damaging transcription factors, oxidative processes can obviously alter gene expression at an early stage and produce dysfunctional proteins downstream that cannot serve their intended purpose in potentially important physiological actions.

In addition to affecting DNA translation and/or transcription, direct oxidation of DNA molecules can occur and produce critical mutations in the genetic backbone itself, again increasing the likelihood of producing abnormal proteins that may adversely affect normal bodily functions. Specifically, proteins that serve as enzymes in key metabolic pathways can undergo changes that neutralize their activity, leading to modified or aberrant actions. Finally, severe derangements in DNA or the proteins it codes for can ultimately result in dysfunctional mitochondria, which, in a vicious cycle, produce more reactive oxygen species, contributing to an ongoing cascade of oxidative damage. If oxidation destruction to the mitochondria is severe enough, the cell can even undergo a process of programmed death or cellular suicide, known as apoptosis, where internal triggers cause the cell to essentially autodestruct.

Examining the adverse effects of oxidative cellular dysfunction even further, contemporary research has demonstrated a clear linkage between redox imbalance and protein functions that could promote cancer propagation. An important discovery in the past few decades that has provided significant insight into the genetic basis of cancer is a gene known as p53. Although originally discovered in 1979, the p53 gene became a centerpiece in scientific journals in the 1990s when mutant p53 genes were reported to be expressed in more than half of human cancers. Further investigation in the early twenty-first century documented the importance of p53 in the stress response of cells.[5] An important protein encoded by the p53 gene is known as the tumor suppressor p53 protein and has been linked to the process of cellular apoptosis, cell cycle arrest (which stops cells from growing out of control as they do in cancer), and cellular aging.[6] Interestingly, research into redox effects on the p53 tumor suppressor protein has demonstrated that oxidative stress can activate key protein factors that interfere with p53 activity and inhibit its ability to stimulate apoptosis, as well as promote microinflammation, cellular transformation, and cellular proliferation—the very processes that define the activities of cancer cells.[7,8] In other words, the p53 gene can be viewed as a regulator that, when functioning normally, is responsible for keeping the system in check and preventing processes from going awry. If this regulator is damaged by oxidative insult, the system breaks down and a host of abnormal activies ensue and lead to cancer cell formation.

In the cardiac arena, ROS-induced injury is a well-documented phenomenon in heart attacks, congestive heart failure, and the promotion of atherosclerosis (cholesterol plaque buildup in the heart arteries). It is well established that both heart failure patients and those undergoing heart attacks have high circulating levels of catecholamines (adrenaline-related substances).[9,10] Studies demonstrate that, when present in excess, catecholamines undergo a process known as auto-oxidation, during which ROS are produced. These toxic particles instigate oxidative destruction that will result in weakened heart muscle and can even contribute to derangements in the electrical activity of the heart that can lead to cardiac arrest.[11-13] Moreover, oxidative modification of cholesterol molecules has been elucidated as a clear pathway in the development of atherosclerosis in coronary artery disease.[14] Without question, processes involving oxidative damage are a clear pathway to the development of both cardiac disease and cancer.

REACTIVE OXYGEN SPECIES IN AGING

Aging is an independent risk for developing numerous conditions, including coronary disease and cancer, as our chances of acquiring such illnesses increases with each decade of life. A discussion of oxidative stress in the aging process, therefore, is apropos to an examination of its effects on the development of cancer and cardiac disease.

In his original 1956 treatise, followed by a more provocative description of mitochondrial function in the aging process in 1972, Denham Harman proposed, in what was known as the "free radical theory of aging," that aging is a result of the accumulated effects of free radical damage to cells over time. Moreover, he principally attributed free radical excess to mitochondrial production or overproduction of reactive oxygen species.[15,16] Since Harman's time, many researchers have implicated a host of cellular byproducts that either directly or indirectly increase ROS concentrations, and multiple lines of investigation have documented a robust linkage between oxidative damage at the cellular level and the aging process.[17-23] Initial studies in animals demonstrated that elderly members of certain species express a greater concentration of ROS than younger members of the same species.[24,25] Additionally, an inverse correlation between the rate of mitochondrial oxidant expression and the maximum life span in different animals has been identified, such that those with greater mitochondrial activity, higher levels of oxygen consumption, and accelerated ROS production demonstrate decreased longevity.[26]

Conversely, other animal studies have shown that genetically altered species who overexpress specific antioxidant enzymes have decreased levels of oxidative damage and demonstrate increased average and maximum life spans.[27] Moreover, caloric restriction in animals, which is known to decrease oxygen consumption and metabolic rate and thereby decrease the production of reactive oxygen species, has been shown to prolong the life span of test subjects.[28-31] Even more, caloric restriction without malnutrition has been shown to reduce protein oxidation, lipid peroxidation, and DNA damage, as well as decrease diseases such as diabetes mellitus and cancer.[28,31] Finally, studies across multiple species, including human beings, has established a positive correlation between maximum life span and activity of the enzyme superoxide dismutase (SOD), which is a critical antioxidant enzyme system that will be discussed later.[26,32]

Animal studies are a provocative foundation for generating hypotheses and providing direction for human research, but what is the actual evidence that oxidative damage exists and is linked to aging in human subjects?

Emanating from Harman's original free radical theory, new investigation has provided deeper insight into the cellular aging process and has even redefined his hypothesis as the "mitochondrial theory of aging," implicating precise intracellular processes that seem to go awry as we get older. The mitochondrial theory holds that mitochondrial DNA, which is present in each mitochondrion within human cells and codes for a multitude of proteins that function within critical energy-producing pathways, undergoes progressive mutations over time. These transformations can occur by exogenous agents such as inhaled or ingested toxins or radiation exposure. Alternatively, transmutations can occur directly via oxidative damage induced by the local production of ROS. Accumulation of these mutations in the mitochondrial DNA then contributes to impaired enzyme production, which, in turn, reduces the function of the mitochondria as aging occurs. Subsequently, the dysfunctional mitochondria further increase the production of ROS, which induce more DNA damage and continue to propagate this vicious cycle.

To add insult to injury, additional evidence suggests that oxidative stress can increase proinflammatory gene expression, resulting in the increased generation of molecules that incite the microinflammatory pathways. Inflammatory mediators can affect a multitude of tissues and organs, and microinflammatory pathways are known to be exaggerated during the aging process. Additionally, the inflammatory cascade has emerged in recent decades as an important mediator of disease processes including arthritis, cancer, cardiovascular disease, and degenerative neurological conditions. The microinflammatory process as it relates to aging and disease will be discussed in detail later.

Recent human investigation has demonstrated age-related mitochondrial malfunction in relation to three fundamental processes: mitochondrial enzyme number and activity, reactive oxygen species production, and ROS-induced oxidative damage. New studies examining the bioenergetics, or functional activity of mitochondria, have clearly shown an age-related decrement in essential mitochondrial enzyme activity. Studies that can "tag" specific mitochondrial enzyme systems have demonstrated marked reductions in key enzyme proteins in heart, diaphragm, and other muscle fibers in aged subjects compared to younger controls. The evidence for human mitochondrial aging and resultant mitochondrial malfunction resides in a multitude of recent studies that have demonstrated that key enzyme pathways within critical organ systems, including the heart, brain, liver, and skeletal muscle, are decreased in number and activity as subjects age. Further, age-related declines in mitochondrial ATP synthesis have also been described in such tissues as skeletal muscle and skin cells.[33-36]

As noted previously, decreases in mitochondrial function are associated with increases in the production of reactive oxygen species, and this correlation is well described in aged human tissues. Additionally, oxidative damage to mitochondrial DNA is well characterized in human beings, and such oxidation-related modifications of mitochondrial DNA have been demonstrated in human heart muscle and diaphragmatic tissue.[37,38] Studies have shown that these DNA defects begin to occur in a host of tissues from individuals in their third decade of life and further accumulate with age. Moreover, cells containing this defective mitochondrial DNA have proved definitively to demonstrate abnormal mitochondrial function, increased levels of ROS, and are more susceptible to stimuli that induce apoptosis.[39,40]

Apoptosis, or the programmed cell death process, is critical to examine in human physiology because its regulation is linked to the process of aging as well as disease development. On one hand, cellular suicide can serve a protective function in preventing cancer cells from multiplying, yet, on the other, it can be responsible for the tissue degeneration that occurs with senescence. Controversy exists regarding the balance of apoptotic processes in aging, but several lines of evidence suggest that cell senescence and programmed cell death are fundamental to the process of aging as well as age-related diseases.

For example, it is well established that age-related cardiac changes include loss of specific heart muscle cells known as cardiomyocytes, and their progressive depletion through apoptotic activity can result in adaptive hypertrophy (thickening) of adjacent cells. This combination clearly correlates with senile cardiac dysfunction that commonly occurs as we age.[41,42] Similarly, apoptosis can occur within brain cells, leading to age-related neurological disorders such as dementia, Alzheimer's disease, Parkinson's disease, and Lou Gehrig's disease.[43] A multitude of investigations have demonstrated similar effects in other tissues, including the liver, reproductive organs, and even blood cells.

The opposite effect appears to occur in cancer development, as age-related oxidative mutations to genes and the proteins for which they code deactivate the apoptosis mechanism. As a result, cellular growth, as opposed to programmed death, occurs because the cellular suicide signals are turned off, allowing cancer cells to proliferate indiscriminately. We will examine more specific mechanisms of cardiac and cancer disease formation in the next sections.

OXIDATIVE STRESS AND CARDIAC DISEASE

The mechanisms of oxidative stress and its resultant effects on different cellular components are well established and have been detailed previously. Following this, it is clear that these processes play a critical role in aging, which, in turn, can contribute to the development of senescent diseases in multiple organ systems. Numerous research studies have implicated oxidative pathways in the formation of different types of cardiac dysfunction, including coronary atherosclerosis and congestive heart failure. We will explore these processes in more detail.

Coronary atherosclerosis involves the process of cholesterol plaque deposition within the walls of the arteries that supply blood to the heart muscle (see figure 3). As the plaque matures, it essentially becomes an amalgamation of an inner core comprised of a soft, viscous, cholesterol-laden pool surrounded by an outer layer of tough, collagen-rich tissue (collagen is an important tissue critical for structural support throughout the body). This dichotomy in the mature plaque is important because the inner layer, if exposed to circulating blood, strongly stimulates the formation of clot, also known as thrombus. The outer layer of tissue, which is known as the fibrous cap, is critically important in containing the cholesterol pool and forming an important barrier between the inner material and the blood flowing through the blood vessel. A "stable" plaque is considered to be one with an intact fibrous cap that disallows the lipid pool to contact the bloodstream. Conversely, an "unstable plaque" is one in which there is disruption in the integrity of the fibrous cap that allows the inner contents to seep out of the plaque and into the bloodstream.

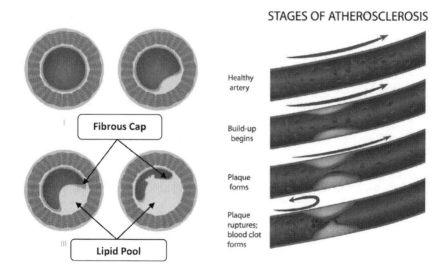

STAGES OF ATHEROSCLEROSIS

Fibrous Cap

Lipid Pool

Healthy artery

Build-up begins

Plaque forms

Plaque ruptures; blood clot forms

Figure 3: Atherosclerosis within an Artery Represented in both cross section and longitudinally, these diagrams depict the progressive accumulation of cholesterol and development of a plaque within the wall of an artery. The large lipid pool is depicted, covered by the often thin fibrous cap. This type of plaque deposition within an artery can lead to heart attack, stroke, and symptoms of peripheral artery disease (PAD).

As the inner and outer layers of the plaque continue to accumulate more material over time, the volume of this atherosclerotic aggregation can expand to the point where it begins to significantly impair blood flow to the heart muscle. This is analogous to the accumulation of debris in the pipes of your sink that eventually cause the water to drain more slowly. If the impairment in blood flow to an individual's heart muscle is significant enough, he or she will begin to experience warning symptoms such as chest pain, known as angina pectoris. In others, angina pectoris does not occur, and instead, their initial manifestation of coronary atherosclerosis will be a heart attack, also known as a myocardial infarction.

During a heart attack, the fibrous cap of an unstable plaque ruptures and causes the contents of the plaque to be exposed to the circulating blood. The lipid material strongly promotes the formation of clot, or thrombus, in the artery in a process known as thrombosis. Eventually, this clot will completely obstruct the vessel and produce complete cessation of blood flow to the heart muscle. If this obstruction is not relieved, the lack of blood flow will cause the heart muscle supplied by the blood vessel to die and, ultimately, may lead to the demise of the patient.

Central to this potentially lethal cascade of events is the process of cholesterol deposition within the wall of the artery. It is well established from research conducted in the 1950s that elevated cholesterol levels are associated with atherosclerosis. Additional investigation in the early 1980s further identified the low-density lipoprotein (LDL) molecule (also known as "bad cholesterol") as the principal culprit in the formation of atherosclerotic plaque. Despite this, however, early research failed to demonstrate the atherogenic effects of LDL particles in test tube experiments, and it wasn't until the late 1980s and early 1990s when researchers discovered that the LDL particle had to be modified prior to exhibiting atherosclerotic properties. The necessary modification, as it turns out, is the oxidation of the LDL particle by reactive oxygen species.

LDL in the blood originates from a molecule produced in the liver known as very low-density lipoprotein (VLDL). VLDL is a complex particle composed of triglycerides, cholesterol, and specific proteins known as apolipoproteins. Once released by the liver into the bloodstream, VLDL interacts with an enzyme in the capillary beds called lipoprotein lipase, which cleaves the triglycerides off of the VLDL molecule, thereby forming the LDL particle.

The circulating LDL molecule can diffuse across the most inner lining of the blood vessel wall, known as the endothelium, which is only a single cell layer thick. Once transported across the endothelium, the LDL particle becomes trapped in what is known as the subendothelial space. It is here where reactive oxygen species, working in concert with other enzyme systems, initiate the process of LDL oxidation.

Once oxidized, these LDL particles aggregate and induce a host of micro-inflammatory reactions that lead to the liberation of constituents known as signaling proteins, which are produced by the endothelial cells. These proteins, in turn, attract a specific type of white blood cell known as the monocyte into the subendothelial space. Monocytes, like most blood cells, are produced by the bone marrow and are a critical component of our immune and inflammatory systems. But how do the monocytes travel through the endothelium into the subendothelial space if the endothelium is supposed to be a protective barrier designed to prevent elements from traversing it?

Simply conceptualized, the endothelium must somehow become more porous, or discontinuous, for the monocyte traversal to occur. In essence, if the endothelium were visualized as a wall, some process would have to occur that would produce holes in the wall for monocytes to flow through. This "hole" is created through a pivotal process in the atherosclerotic cascade known as endothelial dysfunction, which is characterized by an imbalance in the tone, clotting ability, and permeability of this important membrane layer.

A host of disease processes, as well as external factors, can produce endothelial dysfunction. One of the most common external insults is tobacco smoking, which is a strong, independent instigator of aberrant endothelial activity. Additionally, conditions such as diabetes mellitus, high blood pressure, and even high cholesterol itself can provoke malfunction of this important cellular wall. Although the exact mechanisms by which conditions such as tobacco abuse or diabetes mellitus induce endothelial dysfunction are complex, a common thread is the activation of the micro-inflammatory response.

In reaction to specific microinflammatory mediators, the endothelium can become "damaged," causing it to become more porous and allow various cells and other elements to diffuse across it into the subendothelial space. Of critical importance is the transmigration of the monocyte, which, in response to endothelial dysfunction, is readily recruited to sites of micro-inflammatory activation. Once in the subendothelial space, oxidized LDL particles stimulate monocytes to differentiate into scavenger cells known as macrophages. The macrophages, in turn, engulf the oxidized LDL particles and create a new constituent known as the foam cell. This molecule is the hallmark of the atherosclerotic plaque, and as the macrophages continue to engulf more and more oxidized LDL to become mature foam cells, they eventually die, leaving a large cholesterol pool within the subendothelial space. Prior to dying, however, macrophages release a host of signaling proteins of their own that attract supportive smooth muscle cells and stimulate them to secrete substances, including collagen, elastin, and proteoglycans, that form a fibrous matrix. This matrix will eventually cover the cholesterol molecules and becomes the important barrier we previously discussed known as the fibrous cap.

Recall, it is the rupture of this very fibrous cap that leads to the exposure of cholesterol material to circulating blood elements, thereafter stimulating the clotting mechanisms that ultimately obstruct the artery and produce a heart attack. We introduced the concept of the stable and unstable plaque and the fact that the difference between these resides in the integrity of the fibrous cap. Interestingly, the same macrophages that are recruited to the plaque and secrete the substances that form the fibrous cap are also implicated in the eventual destabilization of this important supportive structure! In response to signals that have not been clearly elucidated in laboratory investigations, macrophages will secrete enzymes known as matrix metalloproteinases, collagenases, and gelatinases, which digest the structural components of the fibrous cap, weakening it and making it prone to rupture.

Given the well-defined series of cellular events that result in the formation of the atherosclerotic plaque, it is not surprising that current therapies for atherosclerosis prevention are directed at reducing LDL levels so that these particles cannot be incorporated in the subendothelial space. However, understanding the sequencethat we have just described, there are clearly more steps that can be targeted to further disrupt the formation and maturation of atherosclerotic plaques. Intensive research is currently directed at preventing the seminal event in the atherosclerotic cascade— the oxidation of the LDL particle. We will examine this in detail later as we discuss potential treatments for oxidative stress.

Although much of cardiac research involves atherosclerosis because of its position as the number one killer in this and many other countries, it is important to understand that there are other cardiac conditions that can be affected by oxidative stress. Specifically, it is apparent that other cardiac dysfunctions, such as congestive heart failure (CHF), can also arise from redox imbalance. CHF defines a clinical syndrome in which there is impaired function of the heart muscle either during contraction, relaxation, or both. If there is impairment in the contractile activity of the heart, the patient is said to have a cardiomyopathy, which is essentially a weakening of the heart muscle that results in its inability to effectively pump blood throughout the body. A cardiomyopathy can result from a multitude of insults, including heart attacks, viral illnesses, certain cardiotoxic drugs, and alcohol abuse. Recent studies have suggested a role for increased oxidative stress in the development of CHF irrespective of the causes just described, and the severity of heart failure has been linked to the degree of oxidative stress present in experimental subjects.[47]

One of the key components of the failing heart, regardless of cause, is the development of what is known as adaptive cardiac hypertrophy, or thickening of the heart muscle cells described earlier. In test tube preparations of cardiac cells, hypertrophy can be induced by introducing hormonal or chemical instigators that promote the thickening of the cells. Interestingly, by subjecting cardiac cells to these stimuli, enhanced intracellular ROS production is noted and, more provocatively, can be inhibited by treatment with antioxidants.[48] This certainly suggests a strong role for oxidative stress in the adaptive hypertrophy response and creates a potential target for treatment.

Another characteristic feature of CHF is the impairment in contractile ability of the cardiac myocytes themselves. Like any other muscle in the body, in order to perform correctly, there must be a coordinated and forceful contraction of individual muscle cells working in unison to obtain the final results. Whether the muscle is the bicep being used to pick up a dumbbell or the heart being used to propel blood throughout the body, effective contraction is paramount. Studies have revealed that cardiac cells subjected to ROS demonstrate aberrant contractile function that can be linked to oxidant-related alterations in mitochondrial function, impaired myocardial cell response to calcium (an important element in the contractile apparatus of muscle cells), and dysfunctional calcium cycling and transport within the cell.[48-50]

One of the clearest relationships between oxidative stress and CHF involves a specific drug-induced form of heart failure produced by the chemotherapy agent Adriamycin. This drug has been associated with ROS production, as well as reduced antioxidant reserve, related to depletion in cardiac cells ("antioxidant reserve" refers to a relative excess of antioxidant compounds that are available within our cells used to combat unexpected increases in oxidative stress).[51,52] Moreover, research has demonstrated subjects treated with the antioxidants vitamin E or probucol are less likely to develop Adriamycin-induced toxicity.[53,54] Clearly, in multiple physiological derangements that accompany congestive heart failure, oxidative stress seems implicated and certainly contributes to the insult that results in the cardiac dysfunction.

Whether examining the oxidation of LDL in coronary atherosclerosis or the redox imbalance that occurs in the pathophysiology of congestive heart failure, oxidative stress is a significant component in the development of heart disease. As research better delineates the specific derangements produced by oxidative damage within the heart, a better understanding of the various mechanisms through which reactive oxygen species exert their detrimental effects is being uncovered. Through these revelations, new therapeutic targets and strategies to preventive oxidative damage continue to illuminate the disease management horizon.

OXIDATIVE STRESS AND CANCER

The transformation of normal cells into cancer cells is a complex, multistage process that involves three fundamental stages: initiation, promotion, and progression (see figure 1).[55,56] Oxidative stress is implicated in each of these phases and occurs through the mechanisms already described.

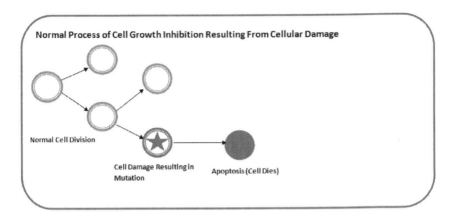

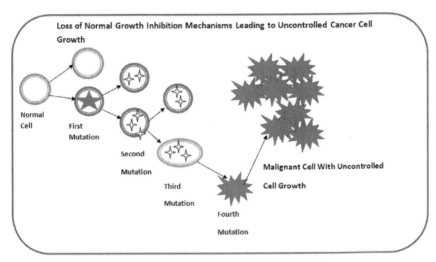

Figure 1: Normal Cellular Mechanisms of Addressing Cellular Mutation versus Cancer Cell Formation In normal cells, a mutation or other cell damage triggers the process of apoptosis, or cellular suicide, thereby eliminating the aberrant cell from the population. In cancer, the initiation phase results from some mutation, but the apoptosis process is blocked. These cells do not look much different than normal cells. This leads to promotion, where additional mutations can occur, causing initial structural changes and functional defects in the cell. Finally, as the cells move to the progression phase, they become structurally distinct and grow uncontrollably.

In the initiation stage, ROS can induce direct DNA damage by creating mutations in the structural DNA components. During promotion, ROS can impair gene expression and produce aberrant redox signaling that results in both enhanced cellular proliferation and reduced cellular apoptosis. Finally, ROS-induced damage can contribute to cancer progression by creating further mutations in DNA within the already dysfunctional cancer cell population.[57]

As described previously, there appears to be incontrovertible evidence that microinflammation instigates cancer production, and recent research has uncovered evidence that links inflammatory processes and cancer transformation to reactive oxygen species. ROS are known to be produced by inflammatory cells that are recruited into regions of tumor growth. This amplification of ROS by microinflammatory mediators can induce further DNA damage and mutation, but also serve to activate signaling pathways that contribute to tumor angiogenesis (a process whereby tumors stimulate the body to produce new blood vessels that are used to supply nutrients to the growing cancer), proliferation, and metastasis.[58-60]

Once cancer cells develop, they must instigate new processes that secure their continued existence. Compared to their normal counterparts, tumor cells are superior in this self-preservation process. By harnessing all of the "natural resources" in their environment, cancer cells monopolize nutrients, blood flow, and other important processes to sustain their own growth. Again, ROS are implicated in the survival mechanisms of tumor cells, as they play critical roles in modulating redox signaling pathways that enhance metabolism within cancer cells and prevent cellular senescence and apoptosis. Additionally, potent enzyme systems can be activated or deactivated through oxidative signaling mechanisms that can promote tumor cell survival as well as down-regulate oxidative defense systems.[61,62]

This combination of effects is much more profound in the cancer cell population and explains how tumors can essentially take over an individual's body over time.

Tumor cell proliferation represents a complex interaction between metabolic and genetic pathways that converge to allow cells to multiply uncontrollably. ROS have been clearly implicated in signaling processes that directly affect the proliferation stage.[63] A fascinating aspect of tumor cell propagation lies in the extensive metabolic requirements that are required to allow cancer cells to multiply. With such an increase in metabolic activity, there is enhanced ROS production, which the tumor cells themselves must attenuate in order to avoid oxidative damage that could produce apoptosis. As a result, sophisticated redox signaling and buffer systems must be employed by proliferating cancer cells in order to prevent their own damage and ensure their growth. Such pathways have been well described and linked to the intricate processes involved in the proliferation of tumors.[64] The fascinating manner in which cancer cells utilize oxidative mechanisms to protect themselves truly underscores the power of the redox system.

Clearly, oxidative stress and redox activity are critical to disease processes such as atherosclerosis and cancer. As we have seen, oxidative stress independently creates a hostile environment that can promote disease through aberrant cellular activity. In the ensuing chapters, however, we will examine how the underlying dysfunction in redox balance is actually instigated by microinflammatory pathways that utilize reactive oxygen species as their foot soldiers to propagate untoward effects within our bodies.

CHAPTER 3:
MICROINFLAMMATION

For most of us, the term "inflammation" conjures images of a swollen, painful joint or a wound that is exquisitely tender, warm, and red. It is an expression that we generally associate with a visible injury, an infection, or a process that occurs following surgery. While this description is accurate, this type of inflammation is considered acute and involves a host of mediators that are activated in response to tissue injury or infection that signal different immune and inflammatory cells to travel to the site of insult. Once at a local site of injury or infection, immune and inflammatory cells attempt to combat the local process by releasing cellular products that are designed to kill microorganisms or assist in repairing the injured tissue. These processes, in turn, are manifested overtly by the consequences we associate with inflammation: redness, swelling, warmth, and pain.

Other times, however, inflammatory and immune pathways are activated at the cellular level, provoked by other processes occurring within us, resulting in changes to our cells and tissues over time that are not noticeable until disease ensues. This chronic inflammation, also known as low-level inflammation or microinflammation, is insidious, does not resolve, and occurs quietly without any clear outward manifestations. Advances in cellular biology and genetic technology have enhanced our ability to examine molecules and processes involved in disease propagation, and new evidence identifies microinflammation as the common link between aging and the development of a multitude of diseases, including cancer and coronary artery disease.

Understanding this connection has fashioned novel arenas for investigation and has delineated new targets in the treatment of underlying risk factors. Most importantly, understanding the microinflammatory basis of disease advances our ability to approach disease prevention, rather than treat diseases after the damage is already done. Indeed, traditional medicine has been deficient in the prevention process, and it has not been until recent decades that preventive medicine has even been considered mainstream in the long-term health maintenance of individuals. Disease treatment, obviously, cannot be abandoned because our most aggressive attempts at prevention will still result in disease development in a certain percentage of the treated population. Nonetheless, prevention should be at the forefront of the comprehensive patient treatment plan.

MICROINFLAMMATION AND CORONARY DISEASE

It wasn't long ago that atherosclerosis was considered a passive process of cholesterol deposition within the artery wall. Early researchers concluded that cholesterol simply "clogged the pipes" over time as the lipid molecules traveled through the bloodstream and eventually found themselves settling in certain blood vessels. Newer insights have clearly identified plaque formation as a complex, active process incorporating the activities of a host of different cell types working in concert to create the atherosclerotic material. It is now well accepted that atherosclerosis is indeed a microinflammatory process that involves a variety of mediators of inflammation, from initiation through progression and ultimately plaque rupture.

As discussed in chapter 2, the initial phase of plaque development involves the migration of monocytes into the vascular wall, followed by maturation of these blood cells into cholesterol-engulfing macrophages. This monocyte is a key participant in the inflammatory process, but different populations of monocytes vary with respect to their microinflammatory properties. Some monocyte populations actually possess low inflammatory activity and contribute to metabolic tissue repair through the activation of growth factors or molecules that stimulate the development of new blood vessels—a key step in many healing processes. Others, however, express receptors that, when stimulated, trigger a complex signaling cascade that results in the production of numerous microinflammatory mediators in addition to reactive oxygen species and protein-cleaving enzymes.[1]

One of the fundamental problems with microinflammation is the fact that it is an unrelenting process that can persist almost indefinitely. Acute inflammation usually abates over a short time, and its resolution is characterized by the evacuation of macrophages and monocytes from inflamed sites. Most of us have readily experienced the acute inflammatory reaction and have witnessed its characteristicmanifestations of redness, warmth, or swelling subside with either specific treatments or simply through the "tincture of time." The perpetual nature of vascular inflammation, however, provides continuous insult within the blood vessel wall and is largely propagated by the continued presence of lipid-laden macrophages within the arterial wall.

Although the process of attracting monocytes to atherosclerotic plaques is well described and highly synchronized, recent investigation has disclosed that the egress of macrophages and other cell populations from tissues is also a tightly regulated process. Interestingly, it appears that high cholesterol itself stimulates macrophages to remain in the vessel wall, and one study has demonstrated that macrophages exposed to normal cholesterol levels will actually migrate out of vascular tissues.[2] Other investigators have identified a molecule called netrin-1 that seems to block the egress of macrophages from inflamed, cholesterol-laden vascular tissue.[3] Whether they are prevented from leaving by netrin-1 or coerced to stay by elevated cholesterol levels,, these cells remain in the vessel wall and contribute to chronic vascular microinflammation and plaque progression.

Eventually, as we previously iterated, the same macrophages that promote chronic inflammation and the development of the atherosclerotic plaque will trigger a sequence of events that will also initiate plaque deterioration. The reasons for macrophages shifting gears and eliciting the plaque destabilization process are elusive. Nonetheless, this process and the resultant plaque rupture occur principally at the local level, with macrophages secreting a host of enzymes that digest the supportive elements of the fibrous cap. In fact, clinical events such as heart attacks are known to occur in atherosclerotic plaques that possess more abundant macrophage concentrations.[4]

Newer evidence also suggests that monocytes circulating in the bloodstream secrete substances that contribute to the plaque destabilization process.[5] Further, another circulating inflammatory white blood cell, called the neutrophil, is known to migrate to sites with inflammatory activity and has also been implicated in the process of cholesterol plaque destabilization and eventual rupture. Neutrophils release their own ROS that produce further lipid oxidation and stimulate the activity of protein-digesting enzymes within the area of the plaque.[6] What was once thought to be an exclusively local process clearly involves a more complex orchestration between different circulating cell lines that work in concert to ultimately produce a destructive and potentially lethal process.

With all of these inflammatory elements converging to create, then destabilize an atherosclerotic plaque, it should come as no surprise that research has identified specific, measurable indicators of microinflammation, known as biomarkers, that are readily detectable in the blood. Such biomarkers can provide us with a glimpse into the microinflammatory activity that is occurring and can be used to predict risk in patients with atherosclerotic disease or other conditions. The most commonly measured inflammatory biomarkers, also known as acute phase reactants, include highly sensitive C-reactive protein (hs-CRP or CRP), serum amyloid A, and fibrinogen. Each of these is produced by the liver in response to substances known as cytokines, which are released by the heart, blood vessel walls, fat cells, and macrophages during inflammatory processes. Commonly measured cytokines include interleukin-1β (IL-1β), interleukin-6 (IL-6), and tumor necrosis factor α (TNF-α). Among the myriad inflammatory biomarkers and cytokines, studies have shown that elevated levels of fibrinogen, a protein that characteristically makes blood sticky, predict risk of long-term death from cardiac causes, and increased IL-6 levels independently predict the risk of heart attack in otherwise healthy male subjects.[7,8] Clinically, however, hs-CRP has been the most extensively studied biomarker and seems to offer considerable utility in risk stratification for individuals with atherosclerotic coronary artery disease.

As noted, hs-CRP is a protein synthesized by the liver that is released in response to inflammatory processes. Obviously, there are many clinical conditions associated with inflammation, so hs-CRP elevations can be nonspecific in the presence of acute inflammatory states. However, in the absence of infection, tissue injury, or chronic inflammatory diseases such as arthritis, hs-CRP elevation is a strong predictor for heart attack, stroke, and cardiovascular death, even when adjusted for traditional risk factors.[10] Studies have demonstrated that hs-CRP adds predictive power to a traditional tool called the Framingham Risk Score, used by physicians to stratify patients into low, intermediate, or high risk categories for sustaining cardiac events (see tables 1 and 2).[11]

Although hs-CRP is useful as a tool to help predict an individual's risk of heart attack, stroke, or death, can it be used to monitor the effectiveness of therapy for cardiovascular disease? Compelling evidence for this has been identified in several clinical trials, most notably the pivotal cardiovascular trials known as CARE, PROVE-IT TIMI 22, and A to Z trials. The CARE

(Cholesterol and Recurrent Events) study demonstrated that treatment with the class of cholesterol-lowering medicines known as statins induces reproducible reductions in hs-CRP levels, independent of its effect on lowering LDL cholesterol.[12] In other words, even though statins potently reduce bad cholesterol levels, they can independently attenuate the microinflammatory response as evidenced by reductions in the inflammatory marker hs-CRP.

PROVE-IT TIMI 22 (Pravastatin or Atorvastatin Evaluation and Infection Therapy-Thrombolysis in Myocardial Infarction 22) had multiple facets of investigation, but notably demonstrated two important effects in coronary disease treatment: (1) the "statin" class of medicines commonly used to treat high cholesterol had a direct anti-inflammatory effect independent of its ability to lower LDL cholesterol, and (2) clinical outcomes were optimum among patients receiving statins who not only achieved low LDL cholesterol levels, but those who reached low hs-CRP levels as well.[13] In other words, PROVE-IT TIMI 22 confirmed the independent antimicroinflammatory effect of statins seen in CARE, but further demonstrated that both low LDL and low hs-CRP independently contributed to good clinical outcomes. This was somewhat groundbreaking data when the prevailing thought at the time was that the clinical benefit of statin therapy was exclusively related to its potency in lowering bad cholesterol levels.

FRAMINGHAM RISK SCORE CALCULATOR			
RISK FACTOR	RISK POINTS (MEN)	RISK POINTS (WOMEN)	POINTS
AGE IN YEARS			
30-34	-1	-9	
35-39	0	-4	
40-44	1	0	
45-49	2	3	
50-54	3	6	
55-59	4	7	

60-64	5	8	
65-69	6	8	
70-74	7	8	
TOTAL CHOLESTEROL			
<160	-3	-2	
160-199	0	0	
200-239	1	1	
240-279	2	1	
$\geq$280	3	3	
HDL CHOLESTEROL			
<35	2	5	
35-44	1	2	
45-49	0	1	
50-59	0	0	
$\geq$60	-2	-3	
SYSTOLIC BLOOD PRESSURE			
<120	0	-3	
120-129	0	0	
130-139	1	0	
140-159	2	2	
$\geq$160	3	3	
DIABETES			
NO	0	0	
YES	2	4	
SMOKER			
NO	0	0	
YES	2	2	
TOTAL POINTS			

Table 1: Framingham Risk Score Calculator Used to determine the relative risk of an individual to develop coronary heart disease (CHD). Based upon different

risk factors, an individual attributes the appropriate number of points for each category. The scores for each category are then combined to achieve a composite Framingham Risk Score. The risk for developing CHD is given in table 2.

10-YEAR CORONARY HEART DISEASE RISK		
POINTS	10-YEAR RISK (MEN)	10-YEAR RISK (WOMEN)
<2	-	1%
-1	2%	2%
0	3%	2%
1	3%	2%
2	4%	3%
3	5%	3%
4	7%	4%
5	8%	5%
6	10%	6%
7	13%	7%
8	16%	8%
9	20%	9%
10	25%	11%
11	31%	13%
12	37%	15%
13	45%	17%
14	53%	20%
15	-	24%
16	-	27%
>17	-	$\geq 32\%$

Table 2: CHD Risk Based Upon Framingham Risk Score The ten-year risk of developing CHD is given based upon the risk score calculated in table 1. Individuals considered low risk have a $\leq$ 10% ten-year risk of CHD, those with intermediate risk have a 10%–20% ten-year risk, and high-risk individuals have a >20% ten-year risk for CHD.

The A to Z (Aggrastat to Zocor) trial was similar to PROVE-IT TIMI 22 in that it assessed the effect of intensive statin therapy in individuals presenting with acute cardiac events. Additionally, it confirmed what was seen in PROVE-IT TIMI 22, such that survivors of cardiac events who achieved lower levels of both LDL cholesterol and hs-CRP derived the greatest clinical benefit.[14] Based upon these and a host of similar trials, hs-CRP appears to be an adequate surrogate to monitor the effectiveness of statin therapy.

To further analyze the utility of microinflammatory biomarkers in risk-stratifying patients, clinical investigation has demonstrated that hs-CRP can help identify individuals who could benefit from aggressive risk factor modification, but do not yet meet accepted criteria for active treatment. Two cornerstone trials have demonstrated a benefit in this regard—the JUPITER trial and the AFCAPS/TexCAPS trial.

AFCAPS/TexCAPS (Air Force/Texas Atherosclerosis Prevention Study) stratified patients without known coronary disease into high and low LDL cholesterol as well as high and low hs-CRP cohorts and followed them longitudinally for an average of 5.2 years. The compelling finding in this study was that individuals who simultaneouslydemonstrated low LDL cholesterol but elevated hs-CRP levels derived a clinical benefit from statin therapy that was identical to the groups who demonstrated high LDL cholesterols.[15] In other words, high levels of the microinflammatory marker hs-CRP was as strong a predictor of the clinical efficacy of statin therapy as the traditional risk factor of high LDL cholesterol.

Similarly, in the JUPITER (Justification for the Use of Statins in Primary Prevention: An Intervention Trial Evaluating Rosuvastatin) investigation, individuals without known cardiovascular disease, lower levels of LDL cholesterol, and elevated hs-CRP levels were prospectively randomized to receive statin therapy versus a placebo and then were followed for occurrence of cardiac and vascular events. In a prospective trial, individuals with specific characteristics are selected in the present and followed into the future while examining the effect of a particular intervention, exposure or other action upon them. All subgroups within the trial were shown to derive a benefit in heart attack, stroke, and the composite of cardiovascular events, including those who would have traditionally been identified as low risk by the Framingham Risk Score.[16] Again, the presence of microinflammation, as evidenced by hs-CRP elevation, identified an at-risk group who would have otherwise been considered lower risk according to traditional criteria. These provocative studies clearly demonstrate that cholesterol is not the only enemy in the atherosclerotic process, and chronic inflammation adds a new dimension for risk stratification and treatment considerations for patients with cardiovascular disease.

Beyond CRP, there is at least one newer microinflammatory biomarker that has demonstrated utility in further stratifying patients with regard to cardiovascular risk. Lipoprotien-associated phospholipase A2, or Lp-PLA$_2$, is an enzyme that works preferentially to cleave oxidized phospholipids such as those found in oxidized LDL particles.[17] Lp-PLA$_2$ is avidly expressed in atherosclerotic plaques and is also found in macrophages residing within the fibrous cap of unstable coronary artery lesions.[18,19] Lp-PLA$_2$ is transported in the bloodstream in association with LDL cholesterol particles, and when it cleaves the phospholipids within oxidized LDL, it produces a proinflammatory and atherogenic byproduct known as lysophosphatidylcholine.[20,21] As a result, serum levels of Lp-PLA$_2$ are generally deemed to correlate with a microinflammatory state, and elevations in this enzyme have demonstrated utility in predicting cardiovascular risk in patients.

One of the landmark trials that demonstrated Lp-PLA$_2$'s association with cardiac risk was known as WOSCOPS (West of Scotland Coronary Prevention Study). This trial was designed to evaluate the use of statins in men with high cholesterol who had not yet had a cardiovascular event. In patients demonstrating the highest levels of Lp-PLA$_2$, there was a twofold increased risk of coronary disease than in those with the lowest levels. Interestingly, CRP was also assessed in this trial, and, similar to Lp-PLA$_2$, the risk associated with the highest levels of CRP was twofold greater than that in subjects with the lowest CRP concentrations.[22] Based upon this, Lp-PLA$_2$ emerged as an independent marker of coronary heart disease.

In another atherosclerosis study known as ARIC (Atherosclerosis Risk in Communities), 12,819 healthy middle-aged men and women were followed longitudinally for over six years in order to determine their risk for developing coronary artery disease based upon Lp-PLA$_2$, CRP, and traditional risk factors. After adjustments for age, sex, and race, individuals within the highest quartiles of Lp-PLA$_2$ and CRP had statistically strong correlation with developing atherosclerotic coronary disease compared to those in the lowest quartiles. Interestingly, CRP and Lp-PLA$_2$ were independently associated with increased risk, but, when taken together at increased levels, the combination of both microinflammatory markers was associated with an almost threefold increase in risk for developing coronary atherosclerosis![23] ARIC confirmed the independent risk prediction seen in WOSCOPS, but provided additional evidence that the predictive powers of CRP and Lp-PLA$_2$ for coronary heart disease are additive. In other words, an individual with either an elevated CRP or Lp-PLA$_2$ level is at increased risk for developing heart disease, but if that same person has elevations in both markers, he or she has a significantly higher risk of developing atherosclerosis.

A subsequent trial known as the MONICA (Monitoring Trends and Determinants in Cardiovascular Diseases) study took ARIC and WOSCOPS one step further and examined cardiovascular event rates as opposed to just the development of atherosclerosis. The MONICA investigators enrolled 934 healthy male subjects between the ages of 45 and 64 with moderately elevated total cholesterol levels and followed their cardiac event rates relative to Lp-PLA$_2$ and CRP concentrations over 14 years. Out of the total population of 934 men, 97 suffered a cardiac event, and their Lp-PLA$_2$

levels were statistically higher than those who did not have an event. Specifically, a robust 23% increased risk for coronary events in those with elevated Lp-PLA$_2$ was identified, suggesting that Lp-PLA$_2$ is not only predictive of atherosclerotic coronary artery disease, but is a marker of future coronary events. Similar to ARIC, the predictive power of Lp-PLA$_2$ was independent of CRP, yet the combination of the two biomarkers powerfully confirmed a statistically significant increase in risk for coronary events, once again suggesting that these two microinflammatory biomarkers may actually be additive in their predictive ability.[24]

Finally, taking Lp-PLA$_2$ beyond coronary atherosclerosis and looking at another manifestation of cardiovascular disease, a study published in 2005 assessed the efficacy of this microinflammatory biomarker in predicting stroke risk. Lp-PLA$_2$ concentration was broken into quartiles and analyzed in 110 stroke victims against a random sample of 1,820 subjects. There was a progressively increased risk of stroke for each higher quartile of Lp-PLA$_2$ level, with the highest quartile demonstrating a 97% increased risk of stroke compared to the lowest![25] Again, the utility of this biomarker in revealing the perils of the microinflammatory state and stratifying at-risk patients is quite provocative, and its ability to signify risk across different manifestations of cardiovascular disease renders it a powerful instrument in the clinician's tool box.

MICROINFLAMMATION AND CANCER

The association between cancer and microinflammation was first recognized by a German physician of the nineteenth century named Rudolf Virchow, who reported that white blood cells—important constituents of the inflammatory response—were usually present in tumor tissue. Subsequent investigation has determined that many different cell populations, as well as chemical mediators associated with immune and inflammatory responses, are concentrated in tumorous regions, further supporting the existence of a link between cancer and inflammation. Epidemiological data has also demonstrated that individuals who use aspirin or a class of anti-inflammatory medicines known as a COX-2 inhibitors have delayed development of premalignant colon tumors known as adenomas. As a result, it is undeniablethat the microinflammatory pathways are intricately linked to cancers, but what is this connection, why does it happen, and how can it be attenuated?

The role of microinflammation in the development of cancer is probably best illustrated by examining well-delineated associations between inflammatory or infectious conditions and certain malignancies. For example, inflammatory bowel disease, a condition characterized by chronic inflammation of the colon or small intestine, is associated with an increased risk of developing colorectal cancer of about 0.5% to 1% per year.[26] Chronic pancreatitis, an inflammatory condition of the pancreas most often associated with alcoholism, is associated with a cumulative risk of developing pancreatic cancer of 1.8% at 10 years and 4.0% at 20 years.[27] Perhaps the most striking example of an inflammatory/infectious process predisposing to cancer development is the human papillomavirus (HPV), which is responsible for virtually all cases of cervical cancer, as well as some cases of anal, vaginal, vulvar, penile, and oropharyngeal malignancy![28-30] The infectious/inflammatory link between HPV and cervical cancer is so provocative, two vaccines have been created specifically against high-risk strains of this virus to protect women against developing HPV-associated cancers. Other examples of inflammatory or infectious-associated malignancies include gastric, ovarian, esophageal, hepatocellular (liver) cancers, Burkitt's lymphoma, and Kaposi's sarcoma. Without question, the microinflammatory link is ubiquitous within the field of oncology and contributes to increased cancer risk for a multitude of patients worldwide.

The concept of cancer-related microinflammation is so pervasive in oncological science that recent investigators have labeled it "the seventh hallmark of cancer."[31] A seminal contribution to cancer biology written in 2000 by Hanahan and Weinberg from the University of California at San Francisco related six original hallmarks of cancer. These are: (1) self-sufficiency in growth signals, (2) insensitivity to antigrowth signals, (3) evading apoptosis, (4) limitless replicative potential, (5) sustained angiogenesis, and (6) tissue invasion and metastasis.[32] Inflammation has developed its place in this scheme largely because two principal pathways of microinflammation, termed extrinsic and intrinsic, have been shown to converge and affect cancer development at all stages. The inflammatory disorders described above represent the extrinsic pathway in which chronic inflammatory states produce mediators and local influences that promote tumor cell formation. The intrinsic pathway refers to largely genetic-driven events that signal cancer cells to express microinflammatory mediators and signals to create a chronic low-level inflammatory milieu within the tumor's microenvironment.

But why does an inflammatory setting promote cancer formation, and where in the cascade is microinflammation active? Similar to research in the atherosclerotic plaque, cancer investigations have revealed that the chronic inflammatory state associated with tumor microenvironments clearly involve the unremitting presence of cytokines, inflammatory cells, and reactive oxygen species. Moreover, recent studies have demonstrated that these inflammatory cells, mediators, or byproducts can activate key transcription factors—proteins that bind to specific DNA sequences that regulate the transfer of information from DNA to messenger RNA—that result in genetic mutations in pathways that normally suppress tumor formation.[33] A transcription factor that we will discover is pervasive in myriad microinflammatory pathways is known as nuclear factor κB, or NF-κB. NF-κB enhances the expression of genes that code for microinflammatory cytokines and contributes to pathways that promote cell survival, cellular proliferation, and new blood vessel formation, or angiogenesis (essential components for tumor cell growth).[34] Therefore, the fundamental physiology behind the coalescence of the intrinsic and extrinsic inflammatory pathways is to create an environment that promotes changes, either genetically or otherwise, that contribute to the very survival of the cancer cells themselves. In essence, through evolutionary "learning," cancer cells beget cancer cells and have developed sophisticated self-preservation mechanisms!

Similar to the atherosclerotic process, there appears to be some clinical utility in assessing microinflammatory biomarkers in cancer. Many of the same markers investigated in the coronary disease arena, including IL-6, TNF-α, and hs-CRP have been examined for clinical applicability in the oncology space. IL-6 has probably been the most extensively studied cytokine, and its dysregulation is known to contribute to many inflammatory disorders.[35] IL-6 also promotes tumor activity in a host of cancer models and has demonstrated some utility in differentiating between individuals with and without malignancies. Moreover, studies have shown that IL-6 levels are directly proportional to the stage and extent of certain malignancies, particularly with regard to colorectal, ovarian, and prostate cancers.[36-38]

TNF-α is not typically produced by noncancerous cells, but malignant ones are known to manufacture it readily. Moreover, it has clearly been linked to the growth and metastasis of various tumors, including pancreatic, skin, ovarian, and colon. TNF-α appears to be important in stimulating new blood vessel formation to help nourish the tumor environment and is known to promote DNA mutation and activation of oncogenes (genes that are implicated in transmitting the information that triggers the formation of cancer cells).[39] From a prognostic standpoint, elevated levels of TNF-α are generally associated with poor outcomes in patients with cancer.

In one study, for example, TNF-α elevations demonstrated a positive correlation with the extent of disease in patients with prostate cancer.[40]

Although their utility is currently being defined, there is evidence to suggest that microinflammatory markers may have clinical application in predicting the extent of disease, monitoring therapy, and even serving as targets for treatment in cancer. Regardless, it is clear that their presence sheds new light on the critical process of chronic inflammation in oncological pathways, and attenuating microinflammation must be a goal in managing cancer risk in patients as well as modulating cancer treatment for those already afflicted.

MICROINFLAMMATION AND AGING

We have already detailed the characteristics of oxidative imbalance that contribute to cellular senescence and the aging process. Examining the redox state further, it is apparent that, in addition to producing direct cellular dysfunction i, redox imbalance associated with aging triggers an increase in the proinflammatory state.[41] As a result, microinflammation, similar to oxidative stress, can be viewed as originating at the cellular level, specifically as a result of dysfunctional mitochondria . The reactive oxygen species produced by these improperly functioning cellular factories, in turn, instigate the microinflammatory pathways. Thus, senescence itself, in the appropriate circumstances, can contribute to the development of a chronic inflammatory state, which, in turn, combined with other risk factors that instigate chronic inflammation, can propagate disease and premature death.

Current research has demonstrated that dysfunctional mitochondria help create a molecular platform known as the inflammasome, which is responsible for activating a host of cytokines and other participants in the microinflammatory cascade. Specifically, the damaged mitochondria will begin to lose their integrity and "leak" molecular components into the cytoplasm (cellular space outside of the mitochondria). Thereafter, proteins that are termed pattern recognition receptors (PRRs), normally expressed by immune/inflammatory cells such as macrophages, monocytes, and neutrophils, detect the leaked mitochondrial contents as harmful and stimulate the formation of the inflammasome complex. This, in turn, triggers the maturation and release of interleukin-1β, which serves to engage and recruit other components of the immune system to destroy the dysfunctional cell.[42] Normally, this cascade is helpful as part of the normal immune response, but, in the case of age-related oxidative damage, it leads to premature cell death, promotes a chronic microinflammatory state, and accelerates the aging process. The formation of the the inflammasome can be viewed as another self-destructive mechanism that can be appropriate under certain circumstances, but detrimental when processes result in premature mitochondrial damage.

Chronic inflammation in the elderly is evidenced by numerous investigations that demonstrate consistently higher serum levels of inflammatory markers such as IL-6 and TNF-α in aged individuals. Elevations in these markers even occur in those elderly individuals with apparently good health and lack of infection.[43,44] It is unclear, however, whether this increase in cytokines and other inflammatory proteins is due simply to senescence, or if other age-related physiological changes are principally responsible. For example, human maturation is generally associated with a relative increase in body fat, and fat cells both produce and secrete IL-6 and TNF-α. In fact, studies demonstrate that fat cells can liberate enough inflammatory mediators to induce a pronounced systemic inflammatory response.[45] More importantly, similar to the process of atherosclerosis, macrophages can infiltrate fatty tissue and continue to propagate the chronic microinflammatory state by releasing their own cytokines. Recent studies have demonstrated that the degree of macrophage migration into the fat tissue is proportional to the body mass index (BMI) of the individual and correlates with the micro-inflammatory response and insulin resistance seen in obese individuals.[46]

In addition to age-related increases in fatty tissue, senescence is associated with decreased levels of the sex hormones, testosterone and estrogen. Interestingly, it is well established that inflammatory cells such as macrophages and neutrophils possess sex hormone receptors that allow these cells to modulate the inflammatory response in various tissues. Moreover, studies have shown that both testosterone and estrogen can suppress the production and secretion of a host of inflammatory biomarkers, including IL-6, TNF-α, and the transcription factor NF-κB.[47-49] It should be no surprise, then, that other investigations have revealed that decreased levels of sex hormones are associated with elevated levels of the same microinflammatory markers.[50] Since levels of both testosterone and estrogen decline with age, their intrinsic propensity to suppress inflammation is reduced, and a chronic low-level inflammatory milieu results.

Regardless of whether aging itself or altered senescent physiological processes are responsible, it is clear that there is an age-related increase in microinflammation. Age-associated obesity can certainly be addressed through fundamental lifestyle modifications to help offset the fat tissue—related contribution to the microinflammatory cascade. Additionally, attempting to maintain hormone balance may be an efficacious therapy, providing the costs and benefits of hormone therapy are appropriately weighed against one another. Most compelling, however, is research targeting the actual microinflammatory and oxidative pathways that produce cell damage and dysfunction, resulting in premature cellular aging and death. .

CHAPTER 4: OBESITY, MICROINFLAMMATION, AND OXIDATIVE STRESS

As we have already discussed, obesity is one of the most modifiable risk factors contributing to both coronary artery disease and cancer. For adults, obesity is defined in terms of a measurement known as the body mass index (BMI), which is calculated from an individual's height and weight (see figure 1). According to the Centers for Disease Control and Prevention, healthy weight is considered to be a BMI between 18.5 and 24.9, overweight is defined as a BMI of 25.0 to 29.9, and obese is considered a BMI of greater than 30.[1] Unfortunately, because of multiple reasons, including poor dietary habits and increased inactivity, obesity has reached epidemic proportions in the United States, with recent reports unveiling a startling 72% overweight or obesity rate for men and a 64% rate for women in this country! Among men, Mexican Americans have the highest prevalence of being overweight or obese at 80%, followed by non-Hispanic whites at 73%, and non-Hispanic blacks at 68%. For women, non-Hispanic blacks had the highest overweight or obesity rate at 78%, followed by Mexican Americans at 77%, and non-Hispanic whites at 61%.[2]

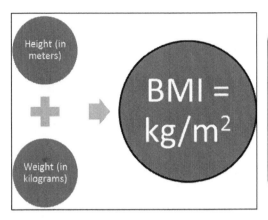

BMI:	Classification
<18.5	Underweight
18.5 - 24.9	Normal Weight
25 – 30	Overweight
30 – 40	Obese
>40	Morbidly Obese

Figure 1: Body Mass Index (BMI) BMI = weight in kilograms/height in meters squared. A majority of Americans exceed a BMI of 25, placing them in the overweight or obese category.

Although Americans are among the most overweight and obese in the world, they are not alone, as the World Health Organization (WHO) reports that since 1980, global obesity has doubled, and 65% of the world's population lives in countries where obesity and being overweight claim more lives than being underweight. According to estimates from 2008 WHO data, over 1.4 billion adults worldwide were overweight, with a startling 500 million individuals being obese![3] These almost incomprehensible statistics undoubtedly delineate a worldwide epidemic for one of the most preventable causes of fatal diseases. Given our remarkable advances in medicine and technology, it is tragic that a condition such as obesity, which can be avoided entirely with lifestyle modifications, continues to contribute so profoundly to worldwide morbidity and mortality!

Perhaps even more disturbing is the fact that corpulence increases the chances of developing other risk factors that further amplify the probability of acquiring diseases such as atherosclerosis and cancer. Obesity unquestionably increases the incidence of another epidemic risk factor, type 2 diabetes mellitus. Data from the Framingham Heart Study demonstrates a doubling in incidence of diabetes over the past three decades, principally among individuals with BMIs greater than 30.[4] Further, multiple epidemiological studies demonstrate that obesity is an independent risk factor for developing high blood pressure, another major risk factor that contributes to the onset and acceleration of atherosclerotic coronary artery disease.[5-8] Finally, both obesity and being overweight contribute to abnormal cholesterol profiles, particularly elevated total and LDL cholesterol, as well as triglycerides.[9] Thus, a vicious cycle ensues with poor dietary and exercise habits contributing to weight gain, which, in turn, increases the likelihood of developing adult-onset diabetes, high blood pressure, and abnormal cholesterol levels. This constellation then increases the chances of developing and propagating diseases such as coronary atherosclerosis and even cancer.

Although the mechanisms through which obesity increase risk factors for coronary disease and cancer have not been clearly elucidated, emerging research visibly identifies obesity's involvement in microinflammation. As described earlier, fat cells, also known as adipocytes, are one of the principal sources of microinflammatory cytokines and serve as the primary storage depot for excess nutrients derived from overeating, underexercising, or both. Adipocyte density increases in response to nutrient excess and, for reasons that are poorly understood, initiate the microinflammatory response to the same stimulus. We shall explore this in more detail.

The initial description of obesity-induced microinflammation occurred in research focused on mouse tissues, where increased levels of TNF-α were discovered in obese mice compared to leaner counterparts.[10] Subsequently, multiple investigations in other animals, as well as humans, revealed that obese subjects express not only increases in TNF-α, but other microinflammatory cytokines such as IL-6 and IL-1β.[11-13] More provocatively, numerous investigations demonstrate that the consumption of specific types of fats is independently associated with a rise in microinflammatory markers. In a study involving young adult and adolescent Asian Indians, intake of saturated fatty acids was the most significant nutrient contributing to elevated hs-CRP levels.[14] Data from another series demonstrated that levels of saturated fatty acids positively correlated with both hs-CRP and fibrinogen.[15] Much attention has been given to eliminating trans fats from our diets, and studies looking at increased trans-fatty acid consumption demonstrate a clear interrelation with elevations in microinflammatory markers, including hs-CRP, IL-6 and TNF-α.[16-18] By contrast, consumption of polyunsaturated fat ("good fat") appears to be inversely associated with hs-CRP, TNF-α, and IL-6 levels , as well as a reduction in another microinflammatory marker known as matrix metalloproteinase 3 (MMP-3).[15,17,19]

Interestingly, parallel lines of research demonstrate that adipocytes are not the only source of these cytokines in obesity. Rather, brain, muscle, liver, and pancreas all increase cytokine expression in states of excess body fat [20-23] Regardless of source, cytokine liberation is clearly related to nutrient excess as well as the consumption of proinflammatory foods. These revelations identify one of the initial microinflammatory processes, and it is quite harrowing to realize that the simple ingestion of unhealthy foods rapidly produces a microinflammatory milieu. Moreover, it is provocative to understand that simple dietary modification can produce as immediate a decrease in measurable inflammatory markers.

In addition to enhanced cytokine expression, obesity is characterized by the increased presence of other inflammatory/immune cells. Studies of adipose tissue during in obese subjectsave revealed increased fatty tissue concentrations of macrophages, mast cells, and another immune cell type known as the natural killer cell.[24-27] The specific activity of these inflammatory/immune modulators has yet to be characterized, but their presence in obesity certainly coincides with microinflammatory activity within the adipocytes, especially given that these cells are the principal liberators of inflammatory cytokines.

Beyond identifying objective markers of microinflammation in obesity, research has demonstrated elevations in related substances—oxidants. We have previously described the intimate relationship between microinflammation and oxidative stress, and this association is readily illustrated by obesity. In one series, for example, glucose and fat intake was positively correlated with not only increases in microinflammatory markers, but elevations in reactive oxygen species as well.[28] Conversely, blood antioxidant levels have been found in consistently lower concentrations in obese subjects compared to their leaner controls.[29-31] Most compelling, research in caloric restriction has demonstrated reductions in both reactive oxygen species and microinflammatory markers in subjects given low-calorie diets or short-term fasting.[32,33] The fascinating interplay between microinflammation and oxidative stress is nicely exemplified by the obese state and certainly explains the foundations for cellular dysfunction that can result from excess body weight. Even more captivating, however, is the prospect that simple caloric restriction can attenuate both microinflammatory and oxidative processes, making this a promising arena for further investigation.

Despite the fact that inflammatory markers and reactive oxygen species are elevated in obese states and during consumption of fatty nutrients and sugar, we have yet to describe what happens physiologically within this microinflammatory, oxidant-rich milieu. In particular, we need to understand what metabolic derangements occur that increase our risk for aging and disease development. It is evident that specific cellular and molecular events do stem from this microinflammatory insult, and we will address these next, focusing on the individual tissue types that have been identified as part of the microinflammatory axis.

During states of nutrient excess, adipocytes increase their accumulation of lipid molecules and expand in size—a process known as hypertrophy. Within these expanding fat cells, microinflammatory mediators have been shown to unequivocally cause insulin resistance, which is the fundamental defect in type 2, or adult-onset, diabetes mellitus. In multiple studies examining the microinflammatory effect in adipocytes, stimulation by TNF-α clearly inhibits glucose uptake through the loss of activity of specific insulin receptors.[34-36] The exact mechanism for this appears to be the activation of specific enzymes that target the insulin receptor. These enzymes create alterations in the receptor that render it incapable of completing the signaling that allows the cell to increase its uptake of sugar. As a result, sugar cannot enter the cells with the dysfunctional receptors, and its concentration increases in the bloodstream, producing the elevated blood sugar levels that define diabetes mellitus.

In addition to inhibiting the insulin receptor, these activated enzymes also stimulate transcription factors such as NF-κB, as well as several others, which further amplify the expression of cytokines and continue to propagate the microinflammatory cascade.[37] As previously described, reactive oxygen species also activate NF-κB and other transcription factors, adding insult to injury in the microinflammatory process. This results in a vicious cycle with persistent, self-perpetuating microinflammation within adipose tissue.

Recall, cytokines produced by fat cells eventually stimulate the liver to produce inflammatory acute phase reactants such as hs-CRP and fibrinogen. CRP levels are increased in individuals with obesity and insulin resistance, and decrease with weight loss, improved insulin sensitivity, and following bariatric (weight loss) surgery.[38-41] The liver functions critically in various cellular pathways, but has noteworthy activity in glucose metabolism as well as the production of fatty acids and cholesterol. It is apparent that obesity increases hepatocyte (liver cell) expression of microinflammatory cytokines and activates inflammatory macrophages within the organ.[42,43] Similar to the process we described in adipocytes, this microinflammatory activation inhibits the insulin receptor signaling cascade within hepato-cytes, preventing normal glucose uptake by these cells.[44] This is significant because the loss of insulin signaling and decreased glucose uptake by the liver results in uninhibited production of glucose by hepatocytes, further exacerbating the already excessive blood sugar levels. In addition to this, liver inflammation induces the production of triglycerides and very low-density lipoproteins (VLDLs), elevating serum levels of these fatty parti-cles, which can then be used to manufacture additional LDL cholesterol.[45] Obviously, enhancing LDL levels increases the concentration of particles that can be oxidized and subsequently incorporated into a new or maturing atherosclerotic plaque.

In addition to these processes, other, local derangements begin to occur in the liver as a response to microinflammatory activation. Interestingly, as chronic low-level inflammation progresses within the liver, a disease known as hepatosteatosis, or fatty liver, can develop. This is most often asymptomatic and detected incidentally during abdominal imaging with ultrasound, CT scans, or MRIs, but, if the microinflammation is allowed to proceed unchecked, it can develop into a more overtly inflammatory condi-tion known as steatohepatitis. This is a perfect illustration of how invisible microinflammation can, and will, eventually cause more explicit and vis-ible "macroinflammation."

Beyond the liver, another critical organ to explore when identifying the metabolic derangements of obesity is the pancreas. As the exclusive source of insulin, and its counterpart glucagon (a hormone that is used to raise blood sugar), the pancreas is critical for maintaining appropriate sugar levels, and its dysfunction creates diabetes mellitus. Of course, it seems obvious that inflammation leading to impaired pancreatic func-tion and decreased insulin secretion would produce type 1 diabetes, but what about obesity and its association with type 2 diabetes? Recent studies have identified that high fat intake increases microinflammatory cytokine expression within the pancreas and promotes the pancreatic accumulation of inflammatory macrophages.[46] Further investigation has shown that during obesity, the increased demand on the pancreas to produce insulin secondary to inflammation-induced insulin resistance essentially overwhelms the insulin-producing pancreatic β cells, causing them to undergo apoptosis.[47] As a result, obesity-induced microinflammation not only produces the insulin resistance that characterizes type 2 diabetes, it instigates pancreatic destruction, producing a relative insulin deficit and further exacerbating the already elevated blood sugars.

Undoubtedly, the pathophysiological derangements resulting from microinflammation are at the heart of the detrimental effects of obesity, but how does all of this cellular dysfunction actually contribute to diseases such as atherosclerosis and cancer? Furthermore, does obesity have any direct effect on the aging process? We will explore these issues next, focusing on the molecular mechanisms at play linking the microinflammation of obesity with senescence and disease development.

OBESITY AND ATHEROSCLEROSIS

Since we have already described the process by which cholesterol plaque is formed, and have elucidated the mechanisms of obesity-induced microinflammation, it is not difficult to postulate how these two processes could intersect. Recall, the formation of the atherosclerotic plaque is a complex interplay of cells, proteins, and other mediators working in microinflammatory and oxidative environs to create a large pool of cholesterol within the wall of the artery. Obesity is characterized by hypertrophy of adipose cells, which subsequently liberate increased amounts of triglycerides and VLDL particles into the bloodstream. Triglycerides are avidly taken up by liver cells that convert them to more VLDL particles. VLDL, in turn, is transformed by enzymes known as lipoprotein lipases into LDL particles that can now be oxidized and incorporated into the cholesterol plaque. Further, via a transfer mechanism not previously described, VLDL actually reduces levels of HDL ("good" cholesterol). Thus, by directly increasing the available LDL substrate and reducing levels of protective HDL, obesity changes the cholesterol balance in favor of promoting the atherosclerotic pathway.

In addition to this, it appears that adipocytes play another role in the atherosclerotic cascade. When we previously discussed the process of plaque development, we introduced the concept that certain proteins are released in chronic low-level inflammatory states and these molecules attract different blood cells to the site of plaque activity. One of these proteins, known as monocyte chemoattractant protein-1 (MCP-1), as the name implies, is responsible for inviting monocytes to the specific plaque development areas. Like a strong magnet attracting iron ore, MCP-1 lures monocytes into the blood vessel walls. These monocytes, in review, transform into macrophages in the presence of oxidized LDL, then engulf those oxidized LDL particles to become foam cells. Eventually, the macrophages die, leaving behind a cholesterol pool that coalesces in the arterial wall. Interestingly, recent studies have determined that adipocytes directly produce MCP-1, and obesity is positively correlated with increased MCP-1 expression in fat cells as well as increased concentrations of MCP-1 in the serum![48,49] As a result, monocyte recruitment is enhanced in those with excess body faty, perpetuating the microinflammatory cascade and stimulating the release of additional MCP-1, which, in turn, recruits additional monocytes into the subendothelial space and directly propagates the atherosclerotic plaque. Again, this nicely illustrates the direct link between obesity-induced microinflammatory insult and the formation of potentially lethal coronary plaques.

OBESITY AND CANCER

Similar to the process of atherosclerosis, oncogenesis, or cancer formation, can be readily linked to obesity. It is well established that increased body mass index contributes to enhanced risk for developing several types of cancer, including esophageal, colorectal, pancreatic, breast, endometrial, kidney, prostate, and gallbladder.[50-52] Moreover, recent data has revealed that obesity is associated with worse clinical outcomes for patients undergoing cancer treatment.[53-56] Although the exact mechanisms for these effects are not completely understood, compelling research has identified specific pathophysiological mechanisms linking obesity to cancer development. There appear to be three primary processes that mediate obesity-related cancers: activity of insulin and insulin-like growth factors, action of protein factors produced by fat cells known as adipokines, and the function of sex hormones.

Based upon a plethora of evidence, insulin and related proteins known as insulin-like growth factors appear to be critical in obesity-related tumorigenesis or cancer cell formation. We have already acknowledged that obesity, by creating insulin resistance, leads to an initial state of insulin excess, or hyperinsulinemia. Insulin-like growth factors are proteins that are chemically similar to insulin that are known to be active in promoting cellular growth as well as inhibiting apoptosis. In research, insulin secretion is often measured by a surrogate marker known as C-peptide, and cancer studies have demonstrated that elevated serum levels of this marker are associated with increased risks of breast, endometrial, and colorectal cancer.[57-60] Further, type 2 diabetes mellitus, independent of obesity, is associated with colorectal, endometrial, pancreatic, and kidney cancers.[61-64] , Insulin excess also appears to stimulate insulin-like growth factor-1 (IGF-1), a protein which has demonstrated proliferative activity that can promote tumor growth.[65] Multiple studies have confirmed a positive correlation between IGF-1 levels and breast, prostate, and colorectal cancers.[66-68] Furthermore,

IGF-1 activation of its specific receptor, IGF-IR, has been shown to produce myriad effects that may instigate tumor growth, including anti-apoptosis, angiogenesis, proliferation, enhanced cell migration, and cell cycle regulation.[69] Despite the decreased insulin receptor sensitivity that occurs with obesity, stimulation of the insulin receptor, as well as the IGF receptor, triggers specific enzyme pathways that are involved in signaling cascades that promote proliferation as well as inhibit apoptosis.[69-71] In other words, the complex actions of insulin and insulin-like growth factors contribute to the fundamental processes that underly cancer cell development.

A second group of protein factors implicated in obesity-related cancer are known as adipokines. Adipokines are a diverse group of protein factors synthesized by fat cells, and the list of new adipokines grows each year as investigators continue to better understand the physiology of adipocytes. To date, there are about fifty adipokines recognized in the literature, but only two are principally implicated in obesity-related cancer: leptin and adiponectin.

Leptin is produced principally by what is known as white adipose tissue. Humans possess two distinct types of fatty tissue: white and brown. Brown fat is generally prevalent in infants, decreasing in concentrations as we become adults, and is used predominantly to generate heat. White fat is the predominant form in adults and is what we normally visualize when we think of the white to yellow substance that accumulates in our abdomen, thighs and other areas. It is often considered its own endocrine organ because in addition to functioning as an energy storage depot, it liberates its own hormones, including leptin and adiponectin.

In addition to white fat, leptin and adiponectin are released in minor concentrations by other tissues, including skeletal muscle, brain, liver, bone marrow, stomach, intestine, and placenta. Leptin's principal physiologic role is to regulate energy intake and outflow by stimulating appetite suppression via a region of the brain known as the hypothalamus. Secondarily, leptin functions in immune regulation, reproduction, glucose metabolism, and inflammation. By stimulating its receptor, leptin activates specific signaling pathways that are involved with cellular proliferation and survival.[72]

Leptin synthesis is influenced by multiple stimuli, including insulin, TNF-α, and sex hormones. Its expression is also increased in hypoxic states (a state of low oxygen that is common in solid tumors). Moreover, serum concentrations of leptin rise in proportion to increased adipose tissue mass, consistent with an obesity-related effect. In cancer cell models, leptin clearly stimulates tumor growth, migration, and proliferation—all pivotal processes in cancer tissue propagation.[73] Further, leptin has an unmistakable link to the microinflammatory pathways, as it has been shown to increase macrophage production of IL-6 and TNF-α.[74] Leptin also reduces tissue sensitivity to insulin, thereby exacerbating the already problematic obesity-related insulin resistance and contributing to more excessive insulin levels. Historic studies have also implicated leptin in the process of angiogenesis, another critical activity in the process of cancer growth and metastasis that involves the formation of new blood vessels to supply nutrients to the enlarging tumor.[75] Finally, leptin upregulates the activity of an enzyme known as aromatase, which is responsible for increasing production of the sex hormone estradiol and promoting tumor growth.[76] This potent constellation of effects certainly demonstrates the pervasive activity of leptin in a wide array of processes that directly stimulate microinflammatory action and promote cancer cell formation and growth.

Shifting from physiology to epidemiology, multiple studies have demonstrated compelling associations between leptin and different types of cancer. Although there is some conflicting data in the literature regarding leptin and breast cancer, one recent observational investigation revealed that leptin and body mass index were positively correlated with tumor stage and classification in postmenopausal women with breast cancer.[77] Further, it appears that in postmenopausal women in whom the principal source of estrogen is adipose tissue, leptin levels correlate with increased breast cancer risk.[77,78] For colorectal cancer, two prospective studies revealed strong correlations between adenomas in men and leptin levels, and one series demonstrated a similar trend in Japanese women.[79-81] There is provocative evidence that thyroid cancer is correlated with obesity, but the association with leptin has only been identified in one study with a specific type of thyroid cancer known as papillary carcinoma.[82-85] In other cancer types such as prostate, esophageal, and endometrial, the link with leptin is less convincing. Nonetheless, there is enough data to suggest that obesity-related leptin elevation contributes to the development of numerous cancer types, certainly substantiating the need for more research in this arena to better clarify this interaction.

Another adipokine, known as adiponectin, has also been the subject of intensive investigation and also appears to correlate with cancer development. Unlike leptin, adiponectin is produced exclusively in adipose tissue and is inversely related to obesity, body mass index, and hypoxia. In other words, increased levels of adiponectin appear to be the norm and actually serve a protective role in inhibiting the process of angiogenesis that tumor cells require for growth. Reduced levels, however, signify a pathological state, and, in addition to the lower concentrations seen with obesity, adiponectin is inversely correlated with microinflammation as well as insulin resistance. Further, studies reveal that both insulin and estrogen can suppress fat cell secretion of adiponectin. Therefore, the metabolic derangements related to adiponectin are evident in states of adiponectin deficiency such as obesity.[86-88]

Whereas there is more controversy in leptin's role in cancer development, studies with adiponectin demonstrate more consistent links between reduced adiponectin levels and cancer development. In breast cancer, decreased circulating concentrations of adiponectin have been associated with increased risk in both pre- and postmenopausal women, with a more consistent inverse relationship in the postmenopausal cohort.[89,90] Similarly, there is a strong inverse correlation between adiponectin levels and endometrial cancer, especially in premenopausal women.[91-94] In colorectal cancer , at least three studies, including the Health Professionals Follow-Up Study, have demonstrated a positive correlation between colorectal cancer and low adiponectin levels.[95-97] Small series have demonstrated similar findings in prostate and gastric cancers, but most other tumor types have shown inconsistent results with regard to adiponectin.[98,99] Although their levels move in opposite directions relative to cancer risk, both leptin and adiponectin concentrations appear to represent important physiological changes that link obesity with tumor propagation. Moreover, this relationship seems to be stronger in certain types of tumors, speaking to the heterogeneous nature of tumor risk, development, and growth.

A final connection between obesity and tumor development appears in the sex hormone, or sex steroid, axis. The principal sex hormone classes in both men and women are androgens and estrogens, of which testosterone and estradiol, respectively, are the principal constituents. Both classes of hormones are derived from cholesterol and produced by both sexes, but the concentration of each hormone is one of the factors that provide sexual differentiation. Estrogen is mainly produced by the ovaries in women, and testosterone is produced chiefly by the testes in men. However, paramount to our discussion of obesity and cancer risk, estrogen can also be synthesized by adipose tissue. An enzyme known as aromatase, or estrogen synthetase, resides in adipose tissue and is responsible for converting circulating testosterone to estradiol. As a result, increased adiposity provides a reservoir for enhanced estrogen synthesis. In turn, the increased risk of breast cancer identified in postmenopausal women is thought to be secondary to a higher rate of conversion of androgens into estrogens through increased activity of the aromatase enzyme system.[100]

Evidence for this heightened sex hormone activity stems from multiple lines of investigation. It is noteworthy that androgen levels are positively correlated with increased adipose tissue in women, providing an increase in available substrate that can be converted into estradiol. However, there may be more to this story, as a meta-analysis of nine prospective studies demonstrated increased breast cancer risk in subjects with elevated concentrations of not only estrogens, but androgens as well. In the same series, increasing body mass index was also positively correlated with breast cancer risk. However, further statistical analysis revealed that this association was essentially attributable to elevated estradiol levels.[101] Elevated breast cancer risk associated with increased serum androgens and estrogens were confirmed in a separate European case-control investigation that examined 677 postmenopausal subjects.[102] Although the exact mechanisms here remain elusive, it is evident that increasing BMI is associated with increased aromatase-related conversion of testosterone to estradiol, and elevation in both of these sex hormones correlates with increased breast cancer risk. Again, the obesity link cannot be ignored in this axis and represents an opportune and relatively simple target to attack in the preventive treatment of tumor development.

Validation for this "simplistic" approach to preventing breast cancer has been assessed in a multitude of studies, dating back to the late 1990s. In a seminal publication from *The New England Journal of Medicine* in 1997, physically active women were found to have a decreased incidence of breast cancer compared to less active controls.[103] Subsequently, data from the Nurses' Health Study, integrating over twenty years of subject follow-up, revealed that postmenopausal women who engaged in the equivalent of nine hours per week of brisk walking had a 15% lower risk of developing invasive breast cancer compared with more sedentary controls.[104] In turn, a new study has confirmed that the combination of diet and exercise resulting in weight loss in postmenopausal women actually reduces both serum estrogens and free testosterone![105] As we demonstrated above, estrogens and androgens are strongly correlated with increases in breast cancer risk, and it is compelling that a simple intervention such as regular exercise and a sensible diet can fundamentally reduce the sex hormone axis that imparts a strong component of the risk for developing breast cancer in women.

Sex hormones also appear to be associated with another cancer in females—endometrial. Traditional risk factors for endometrial cancer include obesity, early initiation of menses, and late menopause—all conditions that are associated with increased longitudinal exposure to estrogens. This observation led to the long-term "unopposed estrogen" hypothesis of oncogenesis, suggesting that cancer risk is related to the duration of exposure to estrogens, which is obviously increased in women who start their menses at an earlier age, experience menopause at a later age, and have increased adipose tissue to convert testosterone to estradiol. In recent decades, obesity-related excess in estrogen has been linked to excess endometrial cell growth or proliferation. Epidemiological studies have also demonstrated that increased estradiol levels not only correlate with endometrial cell development, but also reduced apoptosis and increased expression of IGF-1![106] Recall, under certain conditions, apoptosis is an important mechanism to prevent abnormal cellular growth and IGF-1 has the ability to promote tumor proliferation, so the combination of these two estrogen-induced effects in conjunction with the estrogen-related stimulation in endometrial cell growth creates the perfect storm for cancer cell development. .

There are numerous investigations currently under way assessing the involvement of sex hormones in different types of cancer, but the obesity-related sex hormone linkage appears to be strongest with endometrial and breast tumors. Encouraging is observation in new lines of research that seem to indicate obesity intervention, through diet and exercise, has the potential to reduce cancer risk by shutting down this deleterious hormonal influence. As new information emerges, we hope to better characterize the injurious effects of sex-hormone activity in obese subjects and develop better means of preventing and treating hormone-sensitive tumors.

OBESITY AND AGING

In addition to promoting diseases such as cancer and coronary atherosclerosis, there is growing evidence that obesity independently contributes to the process of premature aging. There are several indicators that support the senescent effect of obesity, but it is largely confined to research on vascular cell lines and a specific component of DNA known as the telomere. We will explore both of these arenas as we elucidate the inescapable impact of obesity on the process of human aging.

Telomeres are specialized DNA structures located on the ends of chromosome strands that do not specifically code for protein sequences. Rather, they function to maintain stability of the DNA structure as they work in concert with other proteins to give the double-stranded DNA molecule structural integrity. Much the way the top platform and side supports of a stepladder help maintain its inverted V configuration, telomeres help the DNA molecule preserve its shape. If the telomere complex is disrupted, this signals the DNA repair system that the DNA strand is "broken," and cellular pathways are activated that will eventually produce premature cellular aging and even programmed cell death.[107]

One of the principal contributors to telomere integrity is their length, and the shorter the telomere gets, the less capable it is of maintaining the structural stability of the DNA molecule. Using the ladder analogy again, imagine how unstable the ladder would become if the top and side supports eroded over time. To a certain extent, telomere shortening is a normal process, particularly during the course of cell replication, where each division leads to a small degree of contraction in the telomere apparatus. Within limits, this can generally occur without any adverse consequence. However, premature erosion of the telomere can decrease its ability to protect the DNA strand, resulting in activation of the DNA repair process described above.

We have previously discussed the deleterious effects that reactive oxygen species can have on lipids, proteins, and other cellular constituents, and it turns out that telomeres are not immune to such insults. In fact, reactive oxygen species have clearly been implicated in the premature shortening of telomeres, which, in turn, incites the cellular aging and apoptosis processes.[108,109] Examination of specific cell lines demonstrates that extended exposure to oxidative stress accelerates telomere contraction in both vascular smooth muscle and endothelial cells, and is associated with shortened telomeres in hypertensive men with elevated serum markers of oxidative stress.[110,111] Conversely, in cell cultures, investigators have revealed that the addition of antioxidants to the culture decreases telomere shortening. These observations strengthen the connection between telomere contraction and oxidative stress.[112]

As we have explored throughout this work, there is an intimate relationship between oxidative stress and microinflammation, with provocative data demonstrating that microinflammation leads the path to cellular destruction. It should come as no surprise, then, that microinflammation is also at the heart of telomere dysfunction! Investigators have demonstrated that elevated IL-6 and hs-CRP levels are associated with decreased telomere length, and, in conjunction with our recent discussion of the sex hormone axis, seems to be more prevalent in postmenopausal as compared to premenopausal women.[113,114]

So it is evident that telomere dysfunction is related to oxidative stress and microinflammation, but how do we make a tighter connection between telomere contraction and obesity? This data was revealed in a study published in 2005, which specifically looked at telomere length in women who were obese and/or smoked cigarettes. In this investigation, it was discovered that telomere length steadily decreased with age across all groups, confirming the age-related telomere contraction that was expected. What was more compelling, and certainly pertinent to our discussion, however, was the fact that there was a statistically significant reduction in telomere length with obese women compared to their leaner controls![115] Subsequent studies have corroborated this, and further investigation has revealed that shortened telomeres are associated with multiple other obesity-related measurements, including elevated body mass index, increased adipose tissue, heightened waist-to-hip ratio, and excess fat accumulation in other organs. Moreover, telomere contraction has been shown to accelerate the already rampant obesity-related aging processes.[116]

In addition to telomere research, investigation into obesity-related activity in the vascular arena has provided some interesting insight into obesity's effect on premature aging. It is well established that senescence involves thickening of the arterial wall and the development of endothelial dysfunction—a process we previously described in which the cells lining the inner wall of blood vessels lose their ability to control the tone, permeability, and regulatory functions of the blood vessels. Recent research spawned by the unfortunate obesity epidemic in children has divulged that such subjects actually demonstrate the same endothelial dysfunction and arterial thickening that normally accompanies their elders, confirming premature senescence at the cellular level![117]

Another striking example of obesity-related endothelial dysfunction involves a critical substance produced by the endothelium known as nitric oxide. Healthy endothelial cells produce nitric oxide, which is a "good" or "helpful" free radical that has many regulatory functions within blood vessels. In obesity, nitric oxide activity is reduced, and this contributes to accelerated rates of atherosclerosis and the development of high blood pressure.[118] Interestingly, studies on aging have demonstrated an identical effect on nitric oxide activity, thereby providing another example of obesity independently inducing a physiological change that is normally present in the senescence.[119]

Persuasive evidence indicates that obesity contributes to cellular and molecular derangements that arise from the microinflammatory pathways and contribute to untoward effects. Whether promoting diseases such as coronary disease and cancer, or accelerating the process of aging, obesity clearly plays a pivotal role in these conditions and induces their appearance at a premature age. As the obesity epidemic worsens in the United States and other countries around the world, it is astounding to realize that by simply bringing body weight back to normal, we can all decrease our likelihood of developing untimely disease and retard the cellular aging process!

CHAPTER 5: DIABETES, MICROINFLAMMATION, AND OXIDATIVE STRESS

One of the biggest challenges facing not only individuals in the United States, but those across the world is the growing prevalence of diabetes mellitus. According to data from the 2011 National Diabetes Fact Sheet published by the American Diabetes Association, 25.8 million children and adults in the United States have diabetes mellitus. Alarmingly, only 18.8 million of these patients are actually diagnosed, leaving 7 million individuals in the US without knowledge of their disease. In addition to this, it is estimated that 79 million people are prediabetic, comprising a population traversing a dangerous path to developing this potentially devastating disease.[1]

For many years, researchers have known that diabetics are often obese, and have generally elevated microinflammatory markers. One of the challenges with independently assessing microinflammation in diabetes is the strong overlap between excess body fat and diabetes mellitus. Based upon our prior discussion of obesity, it should be readily apparent that increased body mass contributes to the diabetic state. Therefore, a discussion of one without the other becomes difficult. Nonetheless, there are some salient features of the microinflammatory state in diabetes mellitus that can be discussed independently of increased adiposity, and we will attempt to focus on these specifically. Additionally, we will endeavor to shed light on the mechanisms by which this destructive disease wreaks havoc on different organ systems and may induce same microinflammatory changes that contribute to conditions such as cancer and atherosclerotic coronary artery disease.

Although most microinflammatory research focuses on type 2 diabetes mellitus, there is some interesting data describing the association between type 1 diabetes mellitus and the inflammatory pathways. In a series examining diabetes progression, those with new-onset type 1 diabetes were found to have CRP levels similar to those seen in healthy controls. However, in individuals with long-term diabetes mellitus, defined as five or more years, CRP levels were significantly higher than nondiabetic controls.[2] This suggests that the microinflammatory process is more insidious, which certainly correlates with the chronic, slowly developing nature of microinflammation that we have previously described. As type 1 diabetics develop complications related to the disease, other studies have demonstrated that there are pronounced increases in microinflammatory and oxidative stress markers, evidenced by elevated levels of IL-Iβ and superoxide anions released by inflammatory cells.[3]

In type 2 diabetes mellitus, intriguing data has revealed that the microinflammatory process, in contrast to that seen in type 1 diabetes, actually seems to precede the development of the disease. Healthy individuals who, in retrospect, are actually in the prediabetic phase, demonstrate increases in microinflammatory markers prior to the development of overt diabetes mellitus.[4-6] This is a fascinating revelation, as such data strongly suggests that the underlying thread in diabetes mellitus is a chronic low-level inflammation that eventually contributes to insulin resistance and dysfunction of the insulin-producing beta cells of the pancreas, ultimately leading to the development of overt diabetes. Moreover, it is compelling that the appearance of microinflammation occurs at different time points in the disease process, depending on whether or not the individual is a type 1 or type 2 diabetic. Although the exact cause of this is unknown, it is possible that the obesity that often precedes type 2 diabetes actually incites the microinflammatory response while the individual is in the prediabetic phase, whereas microinflammation becomes a long-term consequence of type 1 diabetes mellitus.

Other data associating microinflammatory markers with diabetes mellitus date back to the early 1990s, when investigators discovered that the biomarker TNF-α was expressed in the fat cells of obese laboratory animals that demonstrated insulin resistance. Further, by neutralizing TNF-α in these subjects, insulin activity on sugar uptake was improved.[7] As we recounted previously, virtually every microinflammatory marker is expressed in obese animal and human subjects, and there is strong evidence to suggest that the microinflammatory state inhibits normal metabolism and insulin activity. Recall, microinflammatory mediators activate undesirable players such as the transcription factor NF-κB, which leads to cellular dysfunction of insulin-producing cells, their programmed death, and impairment in insulin signaling in insulin-sensitive tissues such as fat cells.

We have not yet discussed in any detail the mechanisms responsible for the development of type 1 diabetes mellitus, but it is worth noting that type 1 disease is mediated by cellular immune reactions in which an individual's own body produces antibodies that attack the insulin-producing beta cells of the pancreas. We have intimated that there is significant overlap between the immune and inflammatory systems, so it should come as no surprise that the activation of this immune response actually instigates the formation of microinflammatory molecules. In turn, this microinflammatory activation appears to promote additional beta cell damage, contributing to further progression of the diabetic state.[8]

In type 2 diabetes, we have described evidence that supports microinflammation preceding the actual diagnosis of the disease. Initial studies assessed nonspecific inflammatory markers such as white blood cell counts and fibrinogen levels—both of which were found to predict the development of type 2 diabetes mellitus.[9,10] Subsequent investigations confirmed that fibrinogen, CRP, and other microinflammatory markers are independent predictors of the development of type 2 diabetes mellitus. In the Insulin

Resistance Atherosclerosis Study (IRAS), serum levels of CRP, fibrinogen, and another microinflammatory marker called plasminogen activator inhibitor-1 (PAI-1) were measured in 1,047 nondiabetic individuals who were then followed for a mean of nearly five years. The chance of a subject converting to diabetes mellitus was assessed and correlated positively with those who had baseline elevations of CRP, fibrinogen, and PAI-1. When corrected for traditional diabetes risk factors, PAI-1 had the greatest predictive power independent of the presence of other risks, whereas the correlation with CRP and fibrinogen was attenuated with adjustment for body fat.[11] Nonetheless, this was powerful evidence supporting the hypothesis that microinflammation is a potent risk for the development of type 2 diabetes.

In another series, over 82,000 women being followed in the Women's Health Initiative Observational Study were prospectively examined with regard to diabetes risk and the presence of the microinflammatory markers TNF-α, IL-6, and hs-CRP. During a median follow-up period of 5.9 years, 1,584 women with diagnosed type 2 diabetes mellitus were analyzed in comparison to a cohort of 2,198 participants who were nondiabetic. Despite adjustment for traditional diabetes risk factors, all three microinflammatory markers were found to be associated with increased risk for developing diabetes mellitus. Again, this provides confirmatory evidence that microinflammation is a predecessor to rather than a byproduct of type 2 diabetes.[12]

In addition to traditional microinflammatory cytokines, adipokines also appear to correlate with the risk of developing type 2 diabetes. Recall, there are numerous adipokines produced by fat cells, with adiponectin being one of the more influential in the obesity and microinflammation arena. This secretory protein has, among many properties, an anti-inflammatory role, and higher levels would be expected to demonstrate a decreased incidence of microinflammatory sequelae such as the development of diabetes. Data from a longitudinal health study on Pima Indians indeed demonstrates an inverse relationship between adiponectin levels and the development of type 2 diabetes mellitus. In fact, those subjects with the highest levels of adiponectin were 37% less likely to develop type 2 diabetes mellitus than those with the lowest concentrations of this anti-inflammatory protein.[13]

In a later study conducted as part of the long-term Atherosclerosis Risk in Communities (ARIC) investigation, adiponectin levels in 10,275 subjects were assessed and similarly correlated with the development of type 2 diabetes mellitus. Again, a strong, graded, and inverse relationship was noted between adiponectin levels and the development of diabetes mellitus, which, when adjusted for other risk factors, demonstrated a robust 40% reduction in risk between those in the highest and lowest quartile of adiponectin concentration.[14] The ARIC study was conducted in both white and African American men and women and demonstrated similar results as the longitudinal Pima Indian health investigation. These data are further corroborated in European, Japanese, and Asian Indian populations, where studies demonstrate similar increases in risk of type 2 diabetes mellitus with decreasing levels of adiponectin.[15-17]

As we have previously noted, microinflammation often creates derangements at the cellular level that also promote the oxidative pathways, and oxidative stress and microinflammation more often than not coexist and propagate one another in a host of disease processes. It appears that diabetes mellitus is not immune in this regard, and there is a plethora of data implicating oxidative stress in the pathophysiology of diabetes. Studies examining typical laboratory surrogates of oxidative stress have repeatedly demonstrated increases in these markers in type 2 diabetics up to five times that of normal subjects.[18-20] Moreover, other investigations have demonstrated that type 2 diabetics possess lower levels of the intracellular antioxidant glutathione, and treatment with standard oral diabetes medicines actually raises the concentration of this important antioxidant.[21,22]

Obviously, the combination of increased oxidative stress with a decreased antioxidant reserve is ominous and would suggest that there would be an objectively quantifiable impact on the cells directly involved in diabetes control. Indeed, a study conducted in the early twenty-first century addressed this topic, specifically examining the difference between oxidative stress-induced damage to the pancreas between diabetic and nondiabetic subjects. Pancreas tissue from diabetic patients demonstrated a significant increase in markers of oxidative stress, as well as a reduction in the expression of antioxidant activity, compared to nondiabetic controls. Moreover, there were statistically significant reductions in beta cell volume and beta cell mass of 22% and 30%, respectively, in the diabetic cohort compared to the nondiabetics.[23] These data confirm that oxidative stress is a critical process in type 2 diabetes mellitus and that there is objective tissue damage that occurs as a direct consequence of imbalanced redox activity within the pancreas.

DIABETES AND CANCER

Given the potent microinflammatory and oxidative milieu created in diabetes mellitus, it should not be surprising that multiple lines of investigation have revealed an association between diabetes and cancer. This is particularly harrowing in view of the worldwide epidemic of diabetes mellitus, as increased rates of this disease raise concern for a potential escalation in cancer development. We have described in detail the interplay between obesity andtumor development and have introduced the concept of obesity-induced insulin resistance as the principal dysfunction promoting obesity-induced diabetes mellitus.. Although most individuals are aware of the intimate relationship between obesity and type 2 diabetes, most are unaware of the strong link between diabetes and cancer, independent of other risk factors, including obesity. We will explore the available evidence in this regard.

Before addressing specific cancers, it is useful to discuss the pathophysiology of diabetes mellitus and its involvement in carcinogenesis. We will focus on type 2 diabetes mellitus, as it is the most prevalent form and represents more than 90%–95% of the cases worldwide. Recall, type 2 diabetes involves a defect in insulin receptor sensitivity, resulting in a compensatory stimulus to increase insulin secretion in an attempt to bombard the receptors and promote the entry of glucose into cells. The hallmark of type 2 diabetes mellitus, therefore, is an excess in both blood sugar and insulin levels—hyperglycemia and hyperinsulinemia, respectively. In type 2 diabetes mellitus, hyperinsulinemia precedes the development of the disease, mirroring the elevation seen with the microinflammatory markers.[24] Insulin excess, in turn, has been shown to affect cancer regulatory processes in both test tube models and actual human studies.

A recently published meta-analysis has revealed that elevated levels of insulin or its byproduct, C-peptide, are clearly associated with an increased risk of developing specific types of cancer, including breast, colorectal, endometrial, and pancreatic.[25] Hyperinsulinemia appears to exert both direct and indirect effects on tumor cells that may promulgate cancer growth. Excess insulin directly stimulates the insulin receptor in tumor cells and appears to promote tumor growth, inhibit apoptosis, and increase chances for cellular invasion.[26] Furthermore, hyperinsulinemia results in activation of the insulin-like growth factor receptor (IGF-1), which is actively expressed in many cancer cells and, when stimulated, induces cellular growth and also inhibits programmed cell death.[27,28] Indeed, excess insulin appears to play a significant role in the mechanism of diabetes-induced increases in cancer formation.

In addition to hyperinsulinemia, researchers hypothesize that hyper-glycemia itself may contribute to oncogenesis. This premise stems from the fact that glucose is a critical nutrient for proliferating cells.[29] Moreover, cancer cells demonstrate a high level of glucose uptake, and research exploring the relationship between glucose concentrations and tumor growth generally demonstrates that tumor cells exhibit higher proliferation rates when exposed to increased glucose levels.[30] Finally, a common characteristic of tumor cells, initially described by the German physiologist and physician Otto Warburg, and appropriately named the Warburg hypothesis, is the observation that cancer cells develop the ability to produce energy from specific metabolic pathways that utilize glucose. This is in contrast to normal cells, which obtain most of their energy from the energy-storing molecule we have previously described known as ATP.[31] As a result, there are sound mechanistic reasons why elevated glucose levels could participate in oncogenesis.

Clinically, numerous investigations have demonstrated that there is a linear rise in risk for cancer with increasing blood sugar levels.[32-35] In the Västerbotten Intervention Project of northern Sweden, correlations between glucose levels and cancer cases were assessed in 33,293 Swedish women and 31,304 Swedish men. Elevated sugar levels were significantly correlated with an increased risk of pancreatic and urinary tract cancer, as well as skin cancer of the malignant melanoma type in both men and women. Moreover, this finding was independent of obesity as measured by body mass index, further strengthening the independent association between hyperglycemia and cancer.[34] Similarly, in an even larger series, the Metabolic Syndrome and Cancer Project (Me-Can), which included cohorts from Norway, Austria, and Sweden consisting of 274,126 men and 275,818 women, data revealed significant increases in incident and fatal cancers of different varieties associated with increased levels of blood glucose. In men, noteworthy increases in risk for multiple myeloma, as well as cancers of the liver, gallbladder, respiratory tract, thyroid, and rectum, were identified. In women, pronounced associations between hyperglycemia and cancer were found for cancers of the pancreas, urinary bladder, uterus, and stomach.[35] Such large series certainly implicate hyperglycemia in the underlying developmentof many types of cancers.

Beyond mechanistic considerations, epidemiological data strongly correlate diabetes mellitus with cancer risk. With regard to breast cancer, it is established that approximately 18%–20% of breast cancer patients have type 2 diabetes.[36] In a large meta-analysis assessing the relative risk of diabetes mellitus with breast cancer, researchers found that the presence of diabetes produced a statistically significant 20% increase in risk of breast cancer in women, as well as a 24% increase in mortality from the disease![37] Similar data were observed in the Swedish Västerbotten Intervention Project, where elevated fasting blood glucose levels were associated with a marked increase in breast cancer incidence.[34] Further confirmation of this association was established in the Nurses' Health Study, which followed 116,488 women for twenty years and demonstrated a 16% increased risk of developing invasive breast cancer in women with type 2 diabetes mellitus.[38]

Perhaps more compelling, and even more alarming, the presence of diabetes portends worse disease and poorer prognosis in women with breast cancer compared to those with normal blood sugars. In a Chinese study assessing breast cancer stage against the presence or absence of diabetes mellitus, the incidence of stage III or stage IV cancer was 41% in the diabetes group, compared to 19% in the nondiabetic cohort.[39] Other series have demonstrated that in patients receiving chemotherapy, those with diabetes mellitus have a 32% greater chance of developing complications compared to those without blood sugar derangements. Moreover, diabetics with breast cancer demonstrate a startling 24%–61% increase in mortality compared to nondiabetics.[40] Clearly, this modifiable, often preventable, risk factor has major implications in the development as well as prognosis of breast cancer that cannot be underestimated.

In addition to breast cancer, pancreatic cancer appears to be strongly associated with type 2 diabetes mellitus. Although pancreatic carcinoma accounts for just over 2% of all malignancies in the world, it is the fourth leading cause of cancer death in the United States.[41] Smoking is the most prevalent risk factor for the disease, with estimates suggesting that about 30% of pancreatic cancer cases are attributable to tobacco use, yet another largely preventable risk factor.[42] In the remainder of cases, the principal instigator of the disease remains elusive. However, multiple series have implicated both obesity and type 2 diabetes mellitus.[43,44]

For example, in a recent meta-analysis assessing the relationship between type 2 diabetes mellitus and pancreatic cancer, researchers examined 36 studies encompassing 9,220 subjects with pancreatic malignancy. In this investigation, an 80% greater risk of pancreatic cancer was identified among individuals with type 2 diabetes mellitus. Interestingly, this association was strongest among individuals with newly diagnosed diabetes, giving critics the opportunity to assert that diabetes is simply an early manifestation of pancreatic cancer, as the risk would be expected to rise with increasing exposure to the diabetes. The counterargument, however, is the fact that those with chronic diabetes mellitus (defined as greater than five years), still possessed a 50% increased relative risk of pancreatic cancer, and, given the highly lethal nature of the disease, it is unlikely that pancreatic cancer would have caused the diabetes so far ahead of its diagnosis.[45] As a result, this meta-analysis certainly provides compelling evidence that diabetes mellitus is more likely a predecessor to pancreatic cancer and may impart significant risk to developing the malignancy.

In addition to this meta-analysis, a case-control study conducted in the San Francisco Bay Area provided further evidence of diabetes as a risk for pancreatic cancer. In this series, 532 case participants were compared to 1,701 controls. Individuals with pancreatic cancer were 50% more likely to report a history of diabetes mellitus than were control subjects. Further, comparing diabetics in the case group with diabetics in the control group, the duration of diabetes was significantly shorter in those with pancreatic cancer, mirroring data observed in the previously described meta-analysis. Similarly, the risk for pancreatic cancer varied with the duration of diabetes, with those having newly diagnosed diabetes (within the previous one to four years) demonstrating a statistically higher risk of developing pancreatic cancer than those with greater than ten years of diabetes mellitus. Further, in individualswith the most severe diabetes, defined as requiring insulin therapy either alone or in combination with oral medications, the risk for pancreatic cancer was 6.8 times higher in subjects using insulin for less than five years compared to those requiring insulin for five or more years.[46] Again, the enhanced risk of short-term versus long-term diabetes in pancreatic cancer is a bit perplexing, and no definitive explanation for this phenomenon has been reached. Nonetheless, the strong relationship between diabetes and pancreatic cancer certainly cannot be ignored.

We have described in detail the microinflammatory basis of colorectal cancer, and it should come as no surprise that, with diabetes mellitus an inciter of microinflammation, colon cancer also ranks among the more prevalent malignancies associated with type 2 diabetes. In a retrospective study conducted in the Rochester, Minnesota, area that followed men and women with clinically confirmed type 2 diabetes mellitus from 1970 to 1994, researchers compared rates of colorectal cancer in their cohort to previously established rates in the Rochester area. Overall, the presence of type 2 diabetes mellitus conferred a 39% increased risk for developing colorectal cancer. Stratified by sex, this risk was exclusively related to the male subjects, where the overall rate of colorectal cancer was 67% higher in patients with diabetes compared to previously established rates in nondiabetics.

Women with type 2 diabetes demonstrated no significant increase in risk for colorectal cancer compared to published rates in the Rochester community.[47]Clearly, the enhanced risk in men was profound, and there is no clear explanation to date for the gender difference. Despite such differentiation, this study certainly provides compelling support for the correlation between diabetes mellitus and colorectal cancer in male subjects.

In a more recent meta-analysis investigating the association between diabetes mellitus and malignancies within the colon and rectum, investigators analyzed 24 studies with a pooled cohort of 3,659,341 participants. Compared to subjects without diabetes mellitus, those with the disease demonstrated a 26% increased risk of developing colorectal cancer. In contrast to the prior study, there was no gender difference in this series, with male and female diabetics demonstrating almost identical risks for developing colorectal malignancies. Another interesting correlation in this meta-analysis was that those subjects receiving insulin therapy (again, a surrogate for more severe diabetes) demonstrated a composite 61% increase in risk for developing colorectal carcinoma.[48] Clearly, in this very large investigation, there is substantial evidence to implicate diabetes mellitus as a risk factor for colorectal cancer, and those diabetics requiring insulin therapy seem to possess an even increased hazard.

In addition to this meta-analysis, other series have examined the issue of whether or not insulin-dependent type 2 diabetes is a more significant risk factor and have yielded similar conclusions. In a retrospective cohort study of patients with type 2 diabetes encompassing 52,872 subjects, insulin use was associated with a greater than twofold risk of developing colorectal cancer. [49] Similarly, in another series, patients with insulin-dependent type 2 diabetes were found to have a threefold increased risk of developing colorectal carcinoma compared to the general population.[50] Finally, in a retrospective study among Korean patients with type 2 diabetes mellitus, colorectal cancer was three times more likely to develop in patients with chronic insulin therapy compared to those not requiring insulin. [51] Without question, the link between diabetes and colorectal cancer is robust, and the presence of worsening diabetes, as evidenced by increased need for insulin, predicts an even greater chance of developing colorectal malignancy.

In addition to colorectal, breast, and pancreatic cancer, diabetes mellitus appears to be a significant risk factor for hepatocellular (liver) cancer. A meta-analysis published in 2006 incorporated twenty-six studies that were diverse with regard to populations and geography. Analysis of data from these multiple investigations demonstrated a composite two-and-a-half-times increased risk of developing hepatocellular carcinoma in diabetic patients compared to nondiabetic controls.[52]

In another investigation conducted as part of the Keelung Community-Based Integrated Screening program in Taiwan, 5,732 diabetic patients out of a total cohort of 54,979 subjects were followed prospectively with the principal goal of assessing their risk for developing hepatocellular carcinoma. Interestingly, this study was conducted in an area with a high prevalence of viral hepatitis infection—an important instigator for the development of liver cancer. After controlling for hepatitis infection, and other risk factors for hepatocellular carcinoma such as alcohol ingestion, investigators determined that individuals with diabetes mellitus possessed a greater than twofold increased risk of developing cancer of the liver compared to nondiabetic controls.[53]

Finally, in a recently published meta-analysis, researchers analyzed forty-nine studies addressing the association between diabetes and hepatocellular cancer. Once again, the presence of diabetes imparted a greater than twofold increase in risk for patients to develop cancer of the liver. Moreover, their results demonstrated an increased mortality rate of nearly two and a half times in patients with hepatocellular carcinoma who were concomitantly diagnosed with diabetes mellitus compared to nondiabetic subjects.[54] These large meta-analyses demonstrate consistent risk profiles over a heterogeneous population with diabetes, providing strong evidence for the link between diabetes and the development of hepatocellular malignancy.

The aforementioned tumor types represent the strongest associations between diabetes mellitus and cancer, but there are a host of other malignancies that also seem to have sound correlations with diabetes. In females, the presence of diabetes appears to be associated with a one and one half to twofold increase in risk for the development of endometrial cancer.[55,56] In kidney malignancies, diabetes appears to significantly increase the chances of developing the cancer by anywhere from 12% to 40%, depending on the population analyzed.[57,58] In non-Hodgkin's lymphoma, a type of cancer of the blood, diabetics have a significant, 12%–41%, increased chance of developing the disease.[59] Other tissue types demonstrate no clear or more controversial associations with diabetes mellitus. Nonetheless, there is an abundance of data supporting the link between diabetes and myriad cancers, and, given the microinflammatory nature of the diabetic state and microinflammation's impact on cancer development and propagation, this should come as no surprise.

Additional perspective on the relationship between diabetes and cancer can be found in studies assessing the effect of diabetes treatment on cancer incidence. In a subsequent chapter, we will discuss, in detail, the antimicroinflammatory properties of a drug used to treat type 2 diabetes mellitus called metformin. This is an oral medication that actually is used for conditions besides diabetes, but has remained at the forefront of type 2 diabetes treatment because of strong efficacy and a good safety profile. Interestingly, as we will describe, the drug has also been found to have potent activity in inhibiting microinflammatory pathways. Given this property, investigators have sought to determine whether treatment with metformin might actually attenuate cancer production and/or propagation.

A meta-analysis published in 2010 provided compelling insight into metformin's activity in this arena. Researchers in Italy compiled data from eleven studies that specifically examined metformin use and cancer incidence or mortality in a composite of 4,042 cancer patients. A statistically significant inverse relationship between both cancer incidence and cancer mortality was noted among subjects taking metformin compared to those taking other diabetes medications. In fact, the risk for cancer development or death was 31% lower in the metformin-treated cohort![60]

Similar observations were disclosed in a meta-analysis conducted by Japanese investigators and published in 2012. In this investigation, researchers pooled data from twenty-four studies involving diabetic sample sizes of 361 to 998,947 patients, comparing cancer incidence and mortality between diabetics taking metformin or not. Their analysis demonstrated that the risk of cancer of any type among diabetics treated with metformin was significantly lower than non-metformin-treated diabetics, with a relative risk reduction of 33%! Further, pooled mortality statistics demonstrated that diabetics with cancer treated with metformin had a 34% reduction in cancer mortality compared to non-metformin users. These two meta-analyses provide compelling insight into the potential for metformin treatment to reduceboth the risk of developing cancer and the chance of dying from cancer.[61] Again, given the known microinflammatory basis of cancer initiation and proliferation, as well as the antimicroinflammatory activities of metformin, this may be a powerful testament to this drug's ability to attenuate diseases other than diabetes!

DIABETES AND CORONARY ATHEROSCLEROSIS

As we have discussed in detail, diabetes mellitus is one of the principal preventable risk factors for developing atherosclerotic coronary disease. According to data from the American Heart Association, heart disease and stroke combined represent the principal causes of death and disability for individuals with type 2 diabetes mellitus. Adults with diabetes have a two- to four-times increased risk of developing heart disease or stroke compared to individuals without diabetes, and about 65% of diabetics will die of some form of cardiovascular disease.[62] These eye-opening statistics are particularly harrowing given the largely avertable nature of type 2 diabetes and certainly highlight the potentially devastating nature of the disease, its public health impact, and the urgent stance we must take in detecting, treating, and, most importantly, preventing it.

Extensive investigation into the mechanisms of diabetes-induced microinflammatory injury to the vascular system has been undertaken over the years to better understand the nature of the number one cause of mortality worldwide, and to find new ways of preventing such devastating consequences. It appears that diabetes mellitus works through a host of mechanisms to exert its injurious effects at the cellular level. The most fundamental derangement appears to be mediated through metabolic by- products that result from the presence of excess glucose. We will explore this now in detail.

A surplus of sugar circulating in the bloodstream initially results in the reversible association of glucose with specific amino acid groups on lipids or proteins. Essentially, because of the sheer excess in sugar molecules, their propensity to bump into and land within "pockets" on lipids or proteins increases. Imagine this interaction in terms of a group of five drinking cups sitting on a table, and a number of ping-pong balls being released above the cups. If there are only a few ping-pong balls released, the likelihood that a majority will make it into the five cups is low. If, however, fifty or one hundred ping-pong balls are released, there is a strong likelihood that each of the cups will house at least one ping-pong ball. Similarly, with large amounts of sugar molecules circulating in the blood, the greater chance there is for random interaction with these open "pockets" on lipid or protein molecules. Once glucose sits in one of these pockets, the resulting molecule is termed an early glycation end product. Those with diabetes mellitus are probably quite familiar with one such early glycation end product known as hemoglobin A_{1c}, which is used by physicians to measure a patient's "average" blood sugar level for purposes of guiding therapy for the disease.

Early glycation end products are generally benign, and, as noted above, can actually be used to help monitor treatment for diabetes mellitus. Remember, at this point, these sugar molecules are not permanently bound to their host lipid or protein particle. Rather, they are loosely associated. In some cases, however, these end products undergo further modification that often involves oxidation, producing a more permanent interaction between the sugar molecule and its host protein or lipid and the development of what are then termed advanced glycation end products (AGEs).[63] Unlike the early glycation end products, AGEs are essentially irreversible once formed and contribute to a host of deleterious effects, both intracellular and extracellular.

Multiple investigations have highlighted the presence of distinct types of AGEs present in high concentrations in blood vessels containing atherosclerotic plaques.[64-66] Moreover, AGE formation has been shown to be accelerated in patients with evidence of oxidative stress and microinflammation. Investigations have also revealed that AGEs are not unique to diabetes and can be produced in response to an oxidative or microinflammatory state instigated by other stimuli.[67,68] As a result, it appears that diabetes mellitus adds insult to injury, with the disease producing a microinflammatory milieu, then propagating it with accelerated AGE production that results from hyperglycemia, microinflammation, and oxidative stress!

So what happens to these AGEs after they form, and why is their presence in atherosclerotic plaques significant? To answer this, we have to discuss

RAGE as opposed to AGE. The receptor for advanced glycation end products, or RAGE, is a molecule that sits on the surface of cells and actually belongs to the immunoglobulin family of protein molecules (immunoglobulins stick out of the surface of cells and are responsible for binding antigens that trigger the immune response).[69] RAGE is minimally present in normal tissues and blood vessels, but has been shown to be abundantly expressed in the blood vessels, endothelial cells, and smooth muscle cells of diabetics.[70,71] The effect of AGEs on cellular activity can be thought of in terms of extracellular and intracellular effects, both of which can hinder normal cell function. When an AGE binds RAGE, the resultant effects are largely intracellular. Conversely, when AGEs exert their effects without binding to RAGE, these are largely extracellular.

Outside the cell, AGEs react with specific molecules in what is known as the basement membrane. The basement membrane is a heterogeneous, very thin layered protein complex that is present in every tissue of the body and is used to scaffold important layers like the endothelium. It can be viewed much like a glue that supports the endothelium and contains multiple constituents, including substances such as collagen, elastin, and laminin, which generally provide structural integrity. AGEs can interact with these proteins and produce what is known as cross-linking between them. As the name implies, cross-linkages involve the binding or union of substances that would otherwise remain independent. Studies of this phenomenon have demonstrated that the specific cross-linkage of collagen to elastin by AGEs results in increased stiffness of the blood vessels.[72,73] Stiffened arteries predispose individuals to the development of high blood pressure and can also accelerate the atherosclerotic process within the arterial walls.

In addition to binding extracellular proteins within the basement membrane, AGEs can also unite with lipids and have even been found to be attached to LDL molecules in both diabetic and nondiabetic subjects.[74] Further investigation has shown that these "glycated" LDL particles, in turn, are less likely to be taken up and cleared from the circulation by normal mechanisms, allowing the LDL particles to circulate longer and increase their likelihood of being incorporated into an atherosclerotic plaque.[74,75] Additionally, AGE-bound LDL particles in diabetics have been associated with decreased nitric oxide production by endothelial cells, resulting in reduced blood vessel relaxation and dilation.[76] Clearly, through extracellular interactions, AGEs are responsible for destructive changes that promote untoward effects on blood vessel structure and function.

In addition to producing undesirable effects outside the cell, AGEs can interact with intracellular proteins and create dysfunction to internal cellular processes. When AGEs attach to RAGEs, studies have shown unequivocal increases in activity of the all-too-familiar microinflammatory transcription factor, NF-κB.[77] Recall, activation of NF-κB induces the transcription of a host of inflammatory cytokines, such as IL-6 and TNF-κ, that propagate the microinflammatory response. Moreover, NF-κB activation increases the genetic expression of other familiar mediators, including vascular cell adhesion molecule-1 (VCAM-1), intercellular adhesion molecule-1 (ICAM-1), and vascular endothelial growth factor (VEGF).[78] Each of these, in turn, contribute in different ways to further exacerbating vascular microinflammation. Combining these intracellular and extracellular effects of AGEs certainly creates a profound diabetes-induced environment ideally suited for propagating the microinflammatory processes that accelerate atherosclerosis.

In addition to these direct actions on the vasculature, AGEs promote other effects that are fundamental to the atherosclerotic process. We have discussed the importance of monocyte migration into the subendothelial space as one of the pivotal activities in the early atherosclerotic cascade.

Studies clearly show that AGEs attract monocytes and actually facilitate their translocation across the endothelial layer into the subendothelial space![79] AGEs have also been shown to induce the genetic expression of LDL receptors on macrophages, the scavenger cells responsible for ingesting the oxidized LDL particles that will form the initial cholesterol plaque within the arterial wall.[80] Finally, AGEs bound to RAGEs are known to stimulate the production of reactive oxygen species, which, in turn, further activate NF-κB and amplify the microinflammatory response. This powerful cascade of events leads to even further augmentation of the already ramped-up atherosclerotic process!

DIABETES AND AGING

Studies assessing the effect of diabetes mellitus on aging are generally sparse. This likely is rooted in our general lack of knowledge of the aging process itself, as well as conflicting hypotheses about the cellular physiology of senescence. Nonetheless, a plethora of observational investigations clearly define similarities between processes associated with both aging and diabetes mellitus. In fact, there are innumerable examples of clinical conditions that occur as a function of both aging and diabetes, provoking many scientists to actually view diabetes as a form of accelerated aging.

One example of this is inherent in the life expectancy of diabetics versus nondiabetics. Studies have shown that, on average, diabetic men and women possess a seven- to eight-year reduction in life span compared to their nondiabetic counterparts.[81] Additionally, age and diabetes mellitus are independent risk factors for the development of cardiovascular disease and its morbid, and often fatal, consequences of heart attack and stroke. Finally, many other clinical conditions are commonly associated with both diabetes mellitus and aging and include impotence, memory loss, increased cancer prevalence, and cataracts.[82-85] These are striking examples of the commonality between aging and diabetes and provide a glimmer of evidence that diabetes mellitus may indeed be a state of premature physiological senescence.

Additional support for the premise that diabetes elicits premature aging relates to the presence of AGEs that we have previously discussed. Recall, the formation of AGEs in diabetes is directly linked to damage within the vascular system. Interestingly, AGEs are not exclusive to diabetics, and studies have demonstrated that aging alone can produce increased AGEs.[86]Additionally, the accumulation of AGEs is accelerated in individuals with poor dietary habits, and increased plasma levels of AGEs are associated with the ingestion of processed foods.[87] As a result, diabetes is not required to produce significant levels of AGEs, and elderly individuals with poor dietary habits are in considerable jeopardy as these toxic products accumulate. Again, this is another illustration of the similarities between aging physiology and the diabetic state.

Possibly the most provocative evidence for diabetes contributing to premature senescence is related to an advanced age surrogate that we have previously discussed known as telomere shortening. Recall, telomeres are specialized regions of DNA that do not code for proteins, but, instead, function to maintain stability of the DNA molecule. Recent research has demonstrated that premature cellular aging is characterized by decreasing telomere length, and, interestingly, studies examining telomere length in patients with diabetes mellitus have demonstrated similar findings. In a recent publication, telomere length was compared between three groups: males with type 2 diabetes of greater than ten years' duration, males with type 2 diabetes of less than one year duration, and healthy male controls. Researchers discovered that both short-term and long-term diabetics had reduced telomere length compared to the healthy controls, with the shortest telomeres present in diabetics diagnosed ten or more years earlier.[88] This compelling data mirrors that seen with both aging and obesity, providing persuasive substantiation that diabetes mellitus may contribute to premature cellular senescence.

Similarly, in a study examining Asian Indian type 2 diabetics, investigators examined not only telomere length, but additional aging surrogates of mitochondrial DNA content and oxidative stress in type 2 diabetics compared to nondiabetic controls. Not surprisingly, statistically significant elevations in oxidative stress markers were found in diabetic subjects compared to controls. Additionally, noteworthy reductions in both telomere length and mitochondrial DNA content were present in those with type 2 diabetes compared to subjects with normal glucose parameters.[89] Again, this is gripping evidence that type 2 diabetes is associated with a multitude of markers of premature aging, further supporting the argument that diabetics are at increased risk for untimely senescence compared to their nondiabetic counterparts.

As we have seen, diabetes mellitus contributes to a host of physiological changes that propagate microinflammatory processes that contribute to cancer, coronary disease, and premature aging. The worldwide epidemic of diabetes is staggering and remains a major public health issue that cannot be ignored, especially given that the overwhelming majority of diabetes is preventable. By opening our eyes to this epidemic and realizing that very simple measures, including diet and exercise, can prevent many cases of diabetes, we can stop the microinflammatory insult it produces and hopefully attenuate the potentially lethal consequences it instigates.

CHAPTER 6: TREATING MICROINFLAMMATION AND OXIDATIVE STRESS—PRIMARY PREVENTION OF AGING AND DISEASE

Since microinflammation results from a complex interaction between our immune and endocrine systems, as well as a multitude of other physiological processes, its treatment must incorporate a multimodality approach to truly achieve prevention. Traditional medical therapies for inflammation have focused on the acute inflammatory diseases and processes such as arthritis or traumatic injury, or after-the-fact treatment once diseases have occurred, leaving a relative void in the conventional management of the microinflammatory state. While there are some compelling therapies available in traditional medicine, focusing exclusively on them is rather myopic since the global preventive therapy for chronic low-level inflammation needs to incorporate four arms: lifestyle modification, chemoprevention, micronutrient supplementation, and nutraceutical administration. We have already discussed lifestyle modification as a focal point in addressing the preventable risk factors, diabetes mellitus and obesity. In this section, we will explore, in detail, the other three facets of microinflammation prevention.

PHARMACOPREVENTION

Pharmacoprevention, also known as chemoprevention, involves the use of traditional medical therapies that have demonstrated evidence-based efficacy in averting disease development. Although most chemopreventive agents are prescription drugs, many of them are not. Before embarking on any individual pharmacopreventive crusade, however, it is important to note that many products, prescription or otherwise, can have significant interactions with other medicines, as well as their own adverse effects. Just because a drug is available over the counter doesn't mean it is either safe or free of significant side effects. The costs and benefits of taking any medicine or supplement should be thoroughly discussed with a physician or other health-care provider prior to its usage.

Aspirin

The most well-studied chemopreventive agent on the market is probably aspirin, which has been used for various ailments since it was originally chewed in the form of willow bark in the fifth century BC. The active ingredient, salicin, was first isolated in the early 1800s and chemically modified to salicylic acid, which was used to treat the inflammatory pain of arthritis. A German chemist named Felix Hoffmann, working for the company Bayer, further modified the salicylic acid compound to acetylsalicylic acid, which eventually became the commercially available drug aspirin, near the beginning of the twentieth century.[1]

As is the case with most medicines, the discovery of aspirin's ability to attenuate cancer risk was discovered incidentally when researchers who were examining colon cancer and precancerous polyps, known as adenomas, realized that individuals with arthritic conditions who were taking regular doses of aspirin had a lower incidence of both adenomas and colorectal cancer. The early part of the twenty-first century marked a new era in our understanding of aspirin's chemopreventive properties, as four independent trials published between 2003 and 2008 definitively proved that aspirin given in doses between 81 and 325 milligrams daily decreased the incidence of recurrent colorectal adenomas.[2-5] This effect was further confirmed, and a dose-response relationship was identified, in another study published by Chan et al. in 2004, which demonstrated that sequential increases in weekly aspirin use provided progressive decreases in the relative risks for developing colorectal adenomas.[6] Although groundbreaking, this news only identified a causal relationship between aspirin and precancerous disease, so researchers set out to answer the question of whether or not aspirin use could actually produce a significant reduction in the true incidence of colorectal cancers.

In a study published in 2005, investigators from the Massachusetts General Hospital provided provocative insights into aspirin's role in attenuating cancer formation in a cohort of over 82,000 women enrolled in a longitudinal health investigation known as the Nurses' Health Study. In this series, researchers determined that individuals taking aspirin for over a decade, at doses of equal to or greater than six 325-milligram tablets per week, had a statistically significant reduction in the incidence of colorectal cancer compared to those who either did not use aspirin or used it infrequently for shorter periods of time. Strikingly, women who ingested more than fourteen adult-strength aspirin tablets per week for more than ten years had a 53% reduction in their risk of developing colon cancer! Of interest, use of other nonsteroidal anti-inflammatory drugs (NSAIDs) demonstrated a similar dose-response effect, with women taking greater than fourteen NSAID tablets per week demonstrating a relative risk reduction in developing colorectal cancer of 46% compared to those taking no NSAIDs! Although this was an exciting revelation in the realm of chemoprevention, significant concerns arose in the incidence of bleeding problems associated with these higher than standard doses of aspirin. It is not difficult to conjecture that the increased use of agents with blood thinning properties might raise the chances of bleeding complications, and, indeed, increased bleeding was noted in this study. As a result, despite a seemingly potent ability to reduce colorectal cancer risk, safety concerns mitigated some of the enthusiasm associated with the pharmacopreventive effects of the drug.[7] Nonetheless, this was groundbreaking information in the realm of pharmacoprevention, demonstrating that an anti-inflammatory agent could have the power to actually prevent the development of at least one type of cancer.

But several questions remained. How could preventive aspirin therapy be applied to general populations considering the potentially harmful doses required to derive maximum benefit? Also, was aspirin only preventive for colon cancers, or could there be a potential effect at attenuating other tumor development? The answer to the dose question was readily within the investigators' grasp because the original studies proving aspirin's benefit in adenoma and colorectal cancer formation clearly demonstrated reduction in risk that actually began at greater than or equal to two tablets per day! In Chan's adenoma study, there was a 14% relative risk reduction in the cohort taking two to five adult-strength aspirin tablets per week, a 32% relative risk reduction for those taking six to fourteen tablets per week, and, finally, the greatest benefit, a 43% relative risk reduction in those taking more than fourteen tablets per week.[6] Similarly, in Chan's cancer study, taking two to five 325-milligram aspirin tablets weekly produced an 11% reduction in the relative risk for developing colorectal cancer, taking six to fourteen tablets produced a 22% risk reduction, and taking more than 14 tablets produced the greatest benefit, with a 32% relative risk reduction![6] Therefore, it was clear that individuals would not have to take excessive doses of aspirin to derive its chemopreventive benefit.

At this point, the critical question of whether or not aspirin could attenuate the development of other cancers remained. Another group of investigators from the United Kingdom set out to unearth the answer by retrospectively analyzing all randomized trials that looked at aspirin and its chemopreventive effects. This investigation examined over twenty-five thousand patients and demonstrated that aspirin actually had a preventive effect in cancers other than those involving the colon. Specifically, it appeared that cancer deaths for all solid tumors during the trial treatment periods in seven trials were reduced after five years of follow-up! At the twenty-year mark, a similar benefit was noted, mostly driven by reductions in cancer deaths from esophageal, colorectal, and lung cancers. Moreover, the benefit was unrelated to aspirin dose (75 milligrams or more), but was more prevalent with age—the greatest benefit being in the group sixty-five years of age and older![8] This provocative new information provides compelling evidence for a pharmacopreventive application of anti-inflammatory therapy as a part of a longitudinal disease-prevention strategy for individuals. Moreover, it provides justification that standard doses of aspirin can confer the chemopreventive effect, thereby at least partially mitigating concerns about its safety profile with regard to bleeding. .

Other beneficial effects of aspirin in chemoprevention are abundant, as studies have shown that this simple drug reduces the activity of key microinflammatory substances, such as the transcription factor NF-κB.[9] Additionally, investigators have shown that aspirin is effective in reducing numerous microinflammatory markers, including hs-CRP, IL-6, IL-1b, and TNF-α.[10,11] Even more provocatively, researchers have identified a new family of molecules called resolvins that are produced from omega-3 fatty acids in response to aspirin therapy and function to combat microinflammatory mediators.[12] Considering the wealth of data available regarding aspirin and colorectal cancer prevention, and the fact that aspirin therapy results in object reductions in microinflammatory indicators, there is significant justification to consider a pharmacoprevention strategy with aspirin, particularly for those with higher risk. Obviously, widespread adoption of aspirin in everybody cannot be justified given the fact that even standard doses of the agent can contribute to bleeding complications. As a result, a pharmacopreventive strategy needs to be discussed with a health-care provider, and the decision to proceed with long-term aspirin therapy needs to be considered in the context of its risk/benefit profile on an individual patient-by-patient basis.

Cyclooxygenase Inhibitors and Other Nonsteroidal Anti-Inflammatory Drugs

Aspirin exerts its effects by inhibiting an enzyme system known as cyclooxygenase (COX). There are two principal COX enzyme systems, termed COX-1 and COX-2, and aspirin irreversibly inhibits both to varying degrees depending on dose. The COX-1 enzyme is responsible for producing moderate amounts of substances known as prostaglandins and thromboxanes. Prostaglandins are fat-derived compounds that mediate a host of physiological responses, including microinflammatory activity, as well as blood clotting action. Thromboxanes are more critically involved in making blood elements known as platelets stick together, not directly exerting any microinflammatory activity. The COX-2 enzyme system is highly expressed in microinflammatory pathways and is responsible for producing large quantities of prostaglandins.

A class of anti-inflammatory drugs known as COX-2 inhibitors, which, as the name implies, selectively inactivate the COX-2 system, has been used for the treatment of arthritis and other acute and chronic inflammatory conditions. Regarding pharmacoprevention, two COX-2 inhibitors, rofecoxib and celecoxib, have been studied in randomized trials, demonstrating efficacy in preventing recurrent colorectal adenomas in individuals with prior histories of these precancerous masses. Although this data is compelling, widespread use of COX-2 inhibitors as a primary prevention strategy has not been adopted because the same trials that demonstrated their efficacy in preventing polyp formation also revealed increased rates of cardiovascular events in the study populations.[13-15] More recently, a pooled analysis of six randomized trials utilizing high doses of celecoxib in non-arthritic patients has revealed no increased cardiovascular risk in individuals with low baseline cardiac risk.[16] This suggests that in appropriate populations who do not possess increased cardiac risk profiles, but who do possess increased risk for development of colorectal cancer, celecoxib therapy may be safely incorporated into a primary prevention treatment strategy.

In addition to aspirin and COX-2 inhibitors, multiple series have demonstrated that other NSAIDs are efficacious in colon cancer prevention. The anti-inflammatory drug sulindac has clearly demonstrated promise in reducing the number of polyps in individuals with an inherited disease characterized by the early development of polyps within the large intestine with a high likelihood of cancerous transformation known as familial adenomatous polyposis (FAP).[17,18] Furthermore, combination therapy with sulindac and an enzyme inhibitor called difluoromethylornithine (DMFO) has demonstrated a 70% reduction in the risk of developing recurrent adenoma.[19]

Beyond colorectal malignancies, extensive investigation has been conducted to determine whether or not NSAIDs demonstrate efficacy in reducing other types of cancers. In a recently e-published study from the periodical *Cancer*, researchers demonstrated that long-term high-intensity therapy with nonselective NSAIDs such as meloxicam, diclofenac, and etodolac is associated with a statistically significant reduction in the development of both squamous-cell and melanoma skin cancers.[20] Given new insights into the inflammatory mechanisms of aging and disease, it is no surprise that aspirin, COX-2 inhibitors, and other NSAIDs have compelling efficacy in suppressing tumor formation. As is always the case in medicine, these, and other drugs, have a risk profile that must be weighed against the potential primary prevention benefits. Considering this, such anti-inflammatory agents may be viable components of a pharmacopreventive regimen in those who have an appropriate cancer risk profile, without excessive hazard for cardiovascular disease, bleeding, or other complications that could be induced by such drugs.

Pentoxifylline

In addition to aspirin, COX-2 inhibitors, and other NSAIDs, a drug named pentoxifylline has demonstrated the ability to modulate microinflammatory effects. Pentoxifylline, which has been available for decades, has been used most extensively as an agent to improve circulation in individuals who have plaque buildup in their leg arteries—a disease known as peripheral arterial disease (PAD). However, recent research has identified potent anti-inflammatory effects of the drug. One study has demonstrated that pentoxifylline attenuates TNF-α signaling, and a more recent trial has shown that treatment with the drug reduces levels of the microinflammatory biomarkers hs-CRP, TNF-α, and fibrinogen.[21,22] Additionally, investigators have discovered that pentoxifylline inhibits the process of leukocyte adhesion, or attachment of white blood cells to the endothelial layer—one of the critical steps involved in atherosclerotic plaque development.[23] Finally, one interesting series has shown that pentoxifylline use for thirty days not only reduces the microinflammatory marker hs-CRP and a measure of active inflammation known as the erythrocyte sedimentation rate (ESR), but it also reduces markers of oxidative stress and increases concentrations of the antioxidant glutathione![24] Yet again, an age-old therapy revisited demonstrates powerful and previously unrecognized effects in microinflammation treatment.

Metformin

Metformin, as we previously introduced, is a drug traditionally used to treat diabetes mellitus that has emerged as another potent inflammatory modulator. Metformin therapy is associated with reductions in hs- CRP, TNF-α, IL-1β, and fibrinogen, with effects seen early, after only thirty days of treatment.[25,26] Further, within twelve weeks of therapy, significant decreases in levels of IL-6 and TNF-α have been observed that rival reductions seen with the two statin agents rosuvastatin and simvastatin.[27,28] Metformin now emerges with a dual impact in treating microinflammation. Principally, it is a critical agent in the treatment of adult-onset diabetes mellitus, reducing the microinflammatory cascade as we discussed during our discussion of diabetes. Now, it secondarily demonstrates promising impact on microinflammatory pathways and adds yet another weapon in the armamentarium against microinflammation and its downstream consequences.

Statins

Perhaps one of the landmark breakthroughs in twentieth-century medicine has been the development of the class of cholesterol-lowering medicines known as statins. Statins, so-called because each drug name ends with "-statin" and is easier to recite relative to their formal name, HMG-CoA reductase inhibitors, have been some of the most well-studied agents in the primary and secondary prevention of coronary disease. In the current practice of cardiology, these agents represent one of the principal weapons against the development and progression of atherosclerotic coronary artery disease. Their efficacy is so potent that many cardiologists almost feel these agents should be "put in the water." Although they are powerful in reducing cholesterol levels and preventing the formation of atherosclerotic plaques, their utility extends event further. Early in their history, it was noted that these medicines possessed a wealth of what are known as pleiotropic effects—actions that occur beyond their primary mechanism. Pertinent to our discussion of microinflammation, one of the well-recognized ancillary effects of statins is their compelling anti-inflammatory activity, which has been demonstrated in a multitude of studies.

Laboratory evidence for the anti-inflammatory effects of statins is abundant in the scientific literature. One study demonstrated that fluvastatin directly inhibits the expression of certain cell surface receptors called CD-11b. This results in decreased adhesiveness of monocytes to the inner lining of blood vessels, which, as we have seen, is an important step before they migrate into the subendothelial space and convert to macrophages that will eventually engulf the LDL cholesterol particles.[29] Another investigation revealed that atorvastatin reduces levels of monocyte chemoattractant protein-1 (MCP-1), which subsequently decreases the activation of the inflammatory transcription factor NF-$\varkappa$B.[30] Further study has demonstrated that treatment with simvastatin for only eight weeks reduces monocyte expression of the microinflammatory biomarkers TNF-α and IL-1β by 49% and 35%, respectively![31] Clearly, there is substantial evidence to support the role of statins in attenuating the microinflammation that characterizes coronary artery and other vascular disease.

But how do the cholesterol medicines produce this anti-inflammatory effect? Although the mechanisms have not been clearly delineated, it is known that statins enhance the activity of certain proteins that, in turn, activate an enzyme known as endothelial nitric oxide synthase (eNOS). This enzyme is primarily responsible for catalyzing the production of substances that control the tone of blood vessels, but it also has been shown to decrease the production of microinflammatory cytokines.[32] By upregulating the activity of eNOS, statins can actually blunt the production of microinflammatory mediators and reduce the degree of low-level inflammation that is occuring.

In the Pravastatin Inflammation/CRP Evaluation (PRINCE) study, patients with and without coronary artery disease wererandomly assigned to receive a placebo agent or the active cholesterol medication, pravastatin, with the primary end point being the change in CRP levels from baseline to twenty-four weeks. During this treatment interval, patients without known coronary disease receiving pravastatin had a median reduction of CRP levels of 16.9%, and actually demonstrated a significant 14.7% reduction in CRP as early as twelve weeks. Importantly, this effect was not correlated with the patients' LDL cholesterol levels, confirming an independent antimicroinflammatory action of the drug.[33]

In a groundbreaking study known as the JUPITER (Justification for the Use of Statins in Primary Prevention: An Intervention Trial Evaluating Rosuvastatin) trial, 17,802 patients with elevated hs-CRP levels, but normal lipid profiles, were randomly assigned to take either a placebo agent or the statin drug, rosuvastatin. JUPITER was unique in that it was the first trial that assessed the effect of cholesterol medicines in patients with normal LDL cholesterol levels and no evidence of coronary artery disease. Patients treated with rosuvastatin demonstrated an average 37% reduction in their hs-CRP levels, but, most provocatively, demonstrated a significant reduction in their risk of heart attack, stroke, and death.[34] These landmark findings provided conclusive evidence that the benefit of statin therapy in attenuating heart attack and stroke risk extends beyond its ability to reduce cholesterol levels, and the decrease in hs-CRP levels corroborate the anti-inflammatory properties of the statin agents.

In addition to the profound role of statins in protecting against the development and progression of atherosclerotic disease, a less publicized effect is their apparent ability to attenuate cancer risk. This observation was initially discovered in several cardiovascular trials when investigators noted a reduced number of cancer deaths occurring in individuals treated in the statin arms.[35] A recent analysis of over three thousand statin users matched to seventeen thousand controls revealed that statins were associated with a 20% reduction in cancer risk, especially in those using the agents longer than four years.[36] In another series, again primarily looking at cardiovascular outcomes, a lower incidence of melanoma skin cancers was noted during analysis of secondary end points.[37] Like many great discoveries, these "incidental" findings provided fascinating insight into a previously unexpected effect of these compounds, and their presence certainly fueled additional investigation into the anticancer effects of statins.

Prospective examination by clinical investigators ensued, and researchers discovered that statins demonstrate activity on a family of intracellular signaling molecules known as Ras proteins. Typically, activated Ras proteins promote appropriate cell growth and differentiation in response to Ras gene stimulation from growth factors. However, when a mutation arises in a Ras gene, Ras proteins can be permanently activated, creating overactive cell division and proliferation independent of the presence of growth factors. As a result, mutant Ras proteins can facilitate cancer growth and differentiation. Statins have been shown to interfere with the activation of Ras proteins, thereby blocking the Ras-related stimulation of tumor growth and maturation.[38] This compelling data suggests that in situations where a Ras gene has mutated and stimulated the overproduction and enhanced activity of growth-promoting Ras proteins, statin therapy may actually be able to keep the Ras proteins in check and blunt the out of control cellular growth response.

Test tube studies identified additional promising effects of statins on two other processes critical to tumor progression: cellular proliferation and apoptosis. In such experiments, statins were shown to both inhibit the proliferative activity of, as well as stimulate apoptosis in, tumor cells from a multitude of cancers, including acute myelogenous leukemia, rhabdomyosarcoma, medulloblastoma, mesothelioma, neuroblastoma, and pancreatic carcinoma. While encouraging, this effect was only seen at very high concentrations of the statin drug, well above the levels that would be observed in patients on standard doses of the agents.[40,41]

Undaunted, researchers continued to probe the utility of statins in the oncology arena, and prospective examinations of statins in standard therapeutic doses did show promise. In a study examining the effect of pravastatin on the survival of patients with advanced liver cancer, those receiving traditional therapy plus a standard 40-milligram dose of the cholesterol drug were compared to a cohort receiving traditional therapy plus placebo. The median survival in the patients receiving placebo was nine months, while the group taking daily pravastatin lived twice as long at eighteen months—a result that reached robust statistical significance.[42] At first glance, this effect may seem somewhat unimpressive given that survival is only extended from nine months to eighteen, but many cancer therapies demonstrate similar results, and an additional nine months of life is important to many patients.

Examining a different tissue type, a nonrandomized study conducted at four community-based centers in the United States assessed the effect of statin therapy relative to breast cancer incidence. The composite cohort consisted of 7,528 women with a mean age of seventy-seven years. Among the individuals taking regular doses of statins, investigators identified an almost twofold reduction in the incidence of breast cancer compared to those not utilizing statin therapy.[43]

Finally, in a population-based, retrospective case-control investigation known as the Molecular Epidemiology of Colorectal Cancer study, 1,953 patients with colorectal carcinoma were analyzed against 2,015 controls without malignancy that were matched by age, sex, and ethnicity. After adjustment for other known risk factors for colorectal cancer, investigators identified a pronounced 47% relative risk reduction in the development of colorectal malignancy in the group utilizing statins for at least five years compared to the nonstatin cohort.[44] Though not definitive, these trials at least support the anticancer potential for statins in three different tissue types of cancer, providing impetus for additional research in this arena.

Although there is promise in many pharmacotherapies for the chemo-prevention of cancer and attenuation of microinflammation, they only form part of the armamentarium against the chronic inflammatory process. In order to truly attack the microinflammatory components of aging and disease, they must be approached from multiple angles and must be tailored to the specific risk profile of each individual. Pharmacoprevention strategies should always be discussed with health-care providers and implemented as part of a comprehensive program to battle microinflammation and its deleterious effects.

TRACE ELEMENTS

Trace elements are minerals we usually obtain from our diets that are physiologically important, but generally only needed in small quantities. The fact that these minerals are required in only minute amounts should not be confused with their significance in our metabolic processes, as most of the trace elements have critical roles in different cellular activities. Most of the time, we obtain trace elements from our diets, but under certain circumstances, individuals do not ingest adequate amounts, or various stressors on our bodies increase our requirements for them. Several trace elements have proven to be significant in the microinflammation arena and show promise in inhibiting chronic inflammatory processes. We will explore these in detail.

Magnesium

Magnesium is perhaps the best-studied trace element, as it has long been known to perform essential roles in a multitude of cellular activities. For example, magnesium is a critical cofactor in nucleic acid synthesis, helping to create the building blocks of our genetic material, DNA. In addition, magnesium is necessary for protein synthesis and is also crucial in the mitochondria during the production of our principal energy molecule, ATP. Magnesium also affects the transport of other ions and, through these interactions, affects the conduction of electrical impulses in the heart, neural impulses in the brain and nerves, and even muscle contraction throughout the body.[45]

It is probably not surprising that magnesium deficiency is relatively common throughout the world, but it may be shocking to realize that nearly 60% of all adults in the United States do not meet the estimated average requirement for magnesium intake![46] Magnesium deficiency, in turn, is correlated with a host of clinical disorders, including diabetes mellitus, high blood pressure, osteoporosis, colon and breast cancer, and atherosclerosis.[46-50] Further, magnesium deficiency has been incontrovertibly shown to have significant activity in microinflammatory pathways, and magnesium-induced microinflammation has been shown to incite oxidative stress mechanisms that result in increased lipid oxidation, reduced antioxidant production, increased concentrations of oxidatively modified proteins, and elevated plasma nitric oxide formation.[45,51]

Multiple studies have demonstrated that magnesium deficiency increases microinflammatory markers, including IL-6 and TNF-α.[51-54] Review of the National Health and Nutrition Examination Survey (NHANES) from 1999–2002 determined that children and adults who consumed less than the recommended daily allowance (RDA) of magnesium were nearly one and a half to two times more likely to have elevated serum CRP levels than those whose magnesium intake was greater than or equal to the RDA.[52,53] In an ethnically diverse cohort of 3,713 postmenopausal women aged fifty to seventy-nine years of age enrolled in the Women's Health Initiative Observational Study, magnesium intake was found to be inversely related to hs-CRP, IL-6, and TNF-α concentrations.[53] Finally, in the Multi-Ethnic Study of Atherosclerosis (MESA) trial, cross-sectional analysis of 5,182 individuals demonstrated a clear inverse relationship between magnesium intake and levels of the inflammatory marker homocysteine.[54] Magnesium is clearly a focal point in the microinflammatory pathways, and inadequate intake of this simple element is unequivocally linked to biomarkers of inflammation.

The association between microinflammatory pathways and oxidative stress has already been described, but magnesium research in redox states further corroborates this important relationship. In multiple series, magnesium deficiency has been linked to microinflammation parameters that, in turn, increase oxidative stress and reduce antioxidant defenses.[55-57] Further, multiple investigations have demonstrated that magnesium deficiency unmistakably produces reactive oxygen species in a variety of tissues, increases oxidant-related tissue damage, elevates the production of superoxide by inflammatory cells, and decreases tissue levels of antioxidants.[59-61] Conversely, sufficient magnesium levels have been shown to prevent reactive oxygen species formation by scavenging free radicals and inhibiting certain enzyme systems responsible for their production.[62] The significance of magnesium in the synergy between microinflammation and oxidative stress cannot be overlooked.

Beyond laboratory findings of inflammation and oxidation, there is a plethora of clinical data that supports magnesium's role in attenuating the microinflammatory response in disease states. The MESA investigators not only elucidated the inverse relationship between magnesium and homocysteine levels, they also discovered that those individuals with the highest intake of magnesium had 24% lower odds of demonstrating atherosclerosis in the carotid arteries![54] In the Women's Health Study, magnesium intake was shown to have a strong inverse relationship with the development of the metabolic syndrome (a combination of risk factors that include obesity, insulin resistance, dyslipidemia, and high blood pressure), with women in the highest quintile of magnesium intake demonstrating a 27% lower risk of developing the syndrome.[63] In a meta-analysis of prospective studies conducted in Stockholm, researchers reported that every 100-milligram increase in magnesium intake decreased the risk of developing type 2 diabetes mellitus by 15%![64] Further, in another series, magnesium supplementation was associated with significant reductions in both systolic and diastolic blood pressures in patients with preexisting high blood presure.[65] Multiple and distinct lines of research testify to the powerful clinical utility of magnesium intake.

In addition to these clinical benefits, there is evidence to suggest that magnesium supplementation may also play a chemopreventive role in cancer. In a large case-control study, total magnesium consumption was positively correlated with a significantly lower risk of colorectal adenoma.[66] Furthermore, two independent investigations revealed that magnesium intake may prevent colon cancer by improving insulin receptor sensitivity in patients who are overweight or have type 2 diabetes mellitus.[67,68] Most recently, a large prospective analysis of over eighty-six thousand Japanese men and women followed for five years in the Japan Public Health Center Study revealed that men in the largest quartile of magnesium intake had a significantly lower risk of developing colorectal cancer compared to those in the lowest quartile of magnesium consumption.[69]

Magnesium's significance in our physiological processes cannot be underestimated, and its relationship to microinflammation and oxidative pathways is critical to understanding how this simple metal can be used to lessen our lifelong burden of chronic low-level inflammation. Moreover, compelling early evidence regarding magnesium's utility in the oncology and cardiovascular arenas provides further impetus for more in-depth research into its protective properties. Adding magnesium and ensuring that our intake meets recommended standards is a simple step toward maintaining an inflammation-free and oxidatively balanced physiological state. This, in turn, can help us battle aging and potentially lethal disease processes.

Selenium

In addition to magnesium, selenium is an important trace element with anti-inflammatory and antioxidant properties. Similar to magnesium, selenium is required for specific cellular functions and is a critical component for key antioxidant enzymes. In selenium-deficient regions of the world, individuals suffer from significantly increased rates of cancer, infections, and inflammatory diseases.[70-72] Although selenium is abundant in a wide variety of food sources such as Brazil nuts, garlic, fish, eggs, and some meats, deficiency can still occur because some foods possess other constituents that can inhibit selenium absorption. Selenium exists in many chemical forms, but most commonly is found in salts such as selenite, selenate, or selenide. In humans, selenium functions are mediated by twenty-five selenoproteins—compounds containing a unique selenium-bound amino acid called selenocysteine.[73]

One of the first selenoproteins to be recognized was glutathione peroxidase, which actually represents a class of enzymes, all of which function in redox reactions to protect cells from oxidative damage. There are currently eight identified glutathione peroxidases, of which four are dependent on selenium for their enzymatic activity. The most abundant version of the enzyme is glutathione peroxidase 1 (GPX1), which is found in almost all mammalian cells and is involved in neutralizing the reactive oxygen species hydrogen peroxide. Other glutathione peroxidases exist in different tissues, or even plasma, and work to protect their respective environments from oxidative stress.[74] The production of glutathione peroxidase is so critical that in states of selenium deficiency, its production is prioritized over that of other selenoproteins.[75]

Another noteworthy selenoprotein in humans and other animals is a family of enzymes known as iodothyronine deiodinases. These proteins are imperative for the activation and deactivation of thyroid hormones, making them a critical regulator of thyroid hormone metabolism. Thyroid hormones are vital to our existence and function principally to regulate our metabolism. Similar to glutathione peroxidases, their activity is dependent on selenium, which is incorporated into the enzymes in the form of an amino acid known as selenocysteine.[76,77]

A third physiologically significant selenoprotein is known as selenoprotein P, or SEPP1. SEPP1 contains ten selenocysteine amino acids and is a significant contributor to plasma selenium levels, making it a good indicator of overall selenium status within humans. It is an important transport protein for the metal and specifically functions to transfer selenium to critical organs, including the liver, brain, kidney, and testis.[78] Further, there is evidence to suggest that SEPP1 functions as a heavy metal chelator, binding toxic metals such as mercury and preventing them from producing harmful effects in our cellular processes.[75]

In order to produce effective selenoproteins, studies have demonstrated that selenium concentrations must fall within strict parameters. On average, selenium concentrations need to be at least 80–90 micrograms per liter (mcg/l) for selenoprotein synthesis and activation to occur. However, maximal glutathione peroxidase activity isn't attained until selenium levels are 100–114 milligrams per liter (mg/l).[79] Given that "normal" selenium levels are considered to be 40–140 mg/l, it appears that the lower normal range would not support maximal enzyme function. It is important to point out, however, that excessive concentrations of selenium, or any trace element for that matter, can produce significant toxicity and adverse events. As a result, it is critical to avoid the "more is better" philosophy when taking trace element supplements.

Considering these reference levels for selenium, multiple studies have demonstrated a significant mortality benefit for those demonstrating higher selenium concentrations. In the US Third National Health and Nutrition Examination Survey (NHANES III), a nonlinear relationship was noted between selenium levels and death from any cause as well as cancer-specific mortality, in over thirteen thousand subjects followed for up to twelve years. In an updated follow-up that extended the observation period to eighteen years, serum selenium levels of 135 mcg/lr or more were associated with reduced mortality.[80] In the Epidemiology of Vascular Ageing (EVA) study, 1,389 elderly French subjects were followed for nine years, and those demonstrating low baseline levels of selenium had a statistically increased mortality risk from cancer.[81] Similarly, in the Baltimore Women's Health and Aging Study, reduced serum selenium concentrations were associated with a significant increase in death from all causes in a five year span.[82]

In addition to these mortality benefits in generalized populations, clinical correlation between selenium concentrations and cancer outcomes has been extensively investigated. In a meta-analysis of sixteen lung cancer studies, higher selenium levels were associated with an overall 26% relative risk reduction in developing lung cancer.[83] Similarly, in a meta-analysis of seven studies analyzing the effect of selenium levels relative to developing bladder cancer, a robust 39% relative risk reduction was identified.[84] In the realm of prostate cancer, results have been more controversial, but at least two meta-analyses have demonstrated a statistically significant reduction in prostate cancer risk in populations with the highest selenium levels.[85,86]

Regarding prospective selenium intake and risk reduction, data from the Nutritional Prevention of Cancer (NPC) trial demonstrated that treatment with daily selenium for four and a half years was associated with a 50% reduction in cancer mortality overall, with significant reductions in the composite incidence of all cancers analyzed as well as independent incidences of , prostate, colorectal, and lung cancers.[87] When re-examined after two more years of follow-up, only reductions in the composite of all cancers and the independent incidence of prostate cancer remained statistically significant.[88] Obviously, more studies in selenium intervention need to be undertaken before routine selenium supplementation can be definitively shown to reduce cancer risk, but these data are compelling and may provide impetus to assess selenium levels and consider supplementation for those at the highest risk.

We have established that selenium is a key cofactor in selenoproteins, at least three selenoproteins have important physiological functions that are essential to life, and selenium levels can predict mortality risk, but what is the evidence that selenium is involved in microinflammatory pathways? A key observation in this regard relates to the finding that decreased concentrations of selenium have been identified in inflammatory states characterized by elevated hs-CRP levels.[89] In another investigation, serum selenium levels, as well as oxidative stress and microinflammatory markers, were assessed in Swedish men at fifty years of age and then repeated twenty-seven years later. Investigators discovered that subjects in the highest quartile of selenium concentration demonstrated the lowest level of both oxidative stress metabolites and cyclooxygenase-mediated microinflammatory markers.[90]

Beyond measuring biomarkers, selenium has been assessed clinically in a host of inflammatory-based conditions. In one study looking at patients with a condition known as severe inflammatory response syndrome (SIRS), selenium supplementation was associated with increased glutathione peroxidase activity and improved clinical outcomes.[91] In a larger multicenter follow-up trial, selenium administration was shown to correlate with reduced mortality in patients suffering from either SIRS or a more severe, and oftentimes lethal, inflammatory syndrome known as septic shock.[92] In an era where so much emphasis is placed on expensive drug therapies including antibiotics, it is compelling to note that significant benefit can be derived from the administration of a fundamental antimicroinflammatory trace element like selenium!

Zinc

Zinc is another trace mineral that is clearly linked to microinflammatory processes. Zinc is the second most abundant trace element in the body after iron and is not stored in any way, making consistent dietary intake of the element essential. Zinc is principally obtained from red meat, but is also present in lamb, seafood, dairy products, yogurt, cereals, and nuts.[93] Zinc deficiency primarily occurs in regions where there is decreased access to animal proteins or increased ingestion of corn and rice, which contain a substance called phytate that prevents zinc absorption.[94] Zinc deficiency is also common among hospitalized patients, particularly the elderly, and is frequently associated with pneumonia, congestive heart failure, and coronary artery disease.[95]

In metabolic processes, zinc is a required cofactor for the activity of over three hundred enzymes![96] In addition, zinc is crucial for the function of multiple key transcription factors involved in signaling pathways, protein synthesis, and the expression of inflammatory cytokines. One vital function of zinc is to inhibit the transcription factor NF-κB, which, as we have previously discussed, is paramount in microinflammatory processes.[97] Recall, NF-κB is critical in the expression of microinflammatory cytokines as well as signaling pathways that control additional inflammatory mechanisms and cellular apoptosis. Suboptimal zinc levels result in suppression of the regulatory proteins that normally inhibit the activity of NF-κB within the cell, thereby increasing NF-κB's proinflammatory action.[98] In other words, when zinc levels are within normal limits, the element enlists the aid of proteins that "guard" NF-κB and prevent it from performing its microinflammatory activity. When zinc levels, drop, however, NF-κB overwhelms its protein guardians and has free reign to exert its effects on inflammatory mediators. Appropriate levels of zinc, therefore, are paramount in the suppression of the microinflammatory state.

Different processes work in concert to modulate our zinc levels, but one fundamental mechanism is through the activity of a family of metal-binding proteins known as metallothioneins. Metallothioneins are small proteins that possess a high affinity for metals such as copper and zinc. Acting similar to a magnet that grabs iron fragments when dragged through the sand, metallothioneins function to sequester metal ions from plasma and tissues, thereby decreasing the availability of free ions to be utilized in other processes. Early research in zinc physiology demonstrated a clear link between the lack of available zinc and impaired immune activity.[99] Further, low zinc availability has been correlated with poor immune function in the aged, as well as increased propensity for the development of age-related diseases.[100]

In acute inflammatory states, zinc sequestration by the metallothioneins increases, and zinc loss in urine and feces is accelerated, leading to further reduction in zinc bioavailability.[101] To make matters worse, microinflammatory cytokines such as IL-6 and TNF-α induce mRNA production of more metallothioneins, increasing the pool of zinc-binding proteins and further decreasing the availability of free zinc ions.[102] Moreover, as chronic inflammation ensues, metallothionein confiscation of free zinc is further accentuated, leading to a greater degree of zinc deficiency.[103] This is yet another example of the many vicious cycles that occur within our bodies as one detrimental process begets another.

It clearly appears that inflammation, whether acute or chronic, induces several pathways that result in decreased zinc levels, but can zinc administration attenuate microinflammatory pathways? In a recently published series, zinc supplementation was compared to placebo in a group of elderly subjects with the primary end points examining this very subject. After six months of therapy, the group taking zinc supplements were found, as expected, to have statistically higher zinc levels compared to the placebo cohort. More importantly, the zinc group demonstrated significantly lower levels of microinflammatory markers, including hs-CRP, IL-6, and MCP-1. Additionally, zinc supplementation was associated with a reduction of other microinflammatory indicators such as serum phospholipase A2 (PLA$_2$), vascular cell adhesion molecule 1 (VCAM-1), and E-selectin. Furthermore, subjects treated with zinc supplements demonstrated decreased lipid peroxidation products and increased antioxidant power, indicating reduced oxidative stress compared to those taking placebo.[104] As a result, this new line of evidence suggests that reduced zinc levels and activity that occurs with microinflammatory insult can be effectively combatted with zinc supplementation.

In another study, women with polycystic ovary syndrome—a condition associated with chronic low-level inflammation—were given zinc supplements versus placebo for a total of eight weeks. Serum levels of zinc, as well as the inflammatory markers hs-CRP and IL-6, were measured pre- and posttreatment. Again, statistically significant elevations in serum levels of zinc were found in the zinc-treated women compared to those taking placebo. Consistent with the previous study, hs-CRP and IL-6 levels were markedly reduced in women taking the zinc supplements, whereas no significant change in microinflammatory markers was noted in the placebo group.[105]

A third investigation assessed the effect of seven weeks of zinc supplementation in healthy elderly subjects, in a nonplacebo-controlled fashion. One unique feature of this trial compared to the previous two was that patients had pre- and posttreatment levels of intracellular zinc measured as opposed to routine serum levels. Additionally, all subjects had pre- and posttreatment assessment of the spontaneous release of the microinflammatory markers IL-6, IL-1β, IL-8, TNF-α, and interferon-Y (IFN-Y). As expected, zinc supplementation was associated with a marked increase in intracellular zinc concentrations that reached statistical significance. Furthermore, striking reductions in the spontaneous release of IL-6 were noted, with posttreatment levels dropping 96.5%! IL-1β levels were reduced by 25.22%, IFN-Y decreased by 10.69%, and TNF-α dropped 3.96%.[106] Based upon these and multiple other trials, there is clear evidence that zinc supplementation has a potent antimicroinflammatory effect as evidenced by these reproducible and unequivocal reductions in microinflammatory biomarkers.

These findings provide compelling evidence that zinc supplementation alone can potently suppress microinflammatory and oxidative pathways, but can this be translated into a more clinically relevant outcome? Zinc's utility in treating patients with myriad illnesses has been examined in the experimental literature, and it is clear that the metal's antimicroinflammatory mechanisms are important in several arenas. One particular area where zinc can be a vital adjunct to patient treatment is in radiation oncology. In one investigation, zinc supplementation was given to patients with head and neck cancers who were undergoing radiation therapy. It is very common for patients receiving radiation treatment for these types of tumors to develop two particular side effects: mucositis and dermatitis. Mucositis is a painful inflammatory reaction to the radiation that involves erosion and ulcer development within the mouth and upper gastrointestinal tract of affected patients. Radiotherapy-induced dermatitis refers to the radiation-associated burn and inflammation that occurs to the skin within the treated area. Approximately 60% of patients receiving radiation treatment for head and neck cancers will develop mucositis, with this rate climbing to 90% if they also have concomitant chemotherapy![107]

Considering the significant rate of side effects to radiotherapy, investigators conducted a randomized trial comparing zinc supplementation to placebo in patients undergoing radiation treatments for their head and neck cancers.

Serum zinc levels were measured in both groups prior to and following treatment, and the time to development and severity of mucositis and dermatitis were assessed during the radiotherapy. Pretreatment zinc levels between the two groups were not different. However, following two months of therapy, there was a pronounced and statistically significant elevation in serum zinc levels in the treatment group compared to placebo. A standard grading system for mucositis and dermatitis derived from the Radiation Therapy Oncology Group was utilized to assign severity of both conditions as grade I, 2, 3, or 4, with grade 4 being the worst. Results of the study demonstrate that grade 2 and 3 mucositis and dermatitis appeared earlier in the placebo group compared to those receiving zinc supplementation. Furthermore, the mean severity grade of the mucositis and dermatitis was lower in those given zinc versus placebo.[108] This is compelling evidence that a simple trace mineral can induce powerful anti-inflammatory activity at the cellular level and help limit the extent of radiation-induced injury occurring on a visible, quantifiable scale!

In another study conducted by the same group of investigators, zinc supplementation was compared to placebo in individuals undergoing radiotherapy for head and neck cancers, but this time the primary end point was patient survival. As expected, the zinc levels following treatment were statistically higher in the group receiving zinc supplements. Although the overall rates of survival were similar between the two groups, the researchers discovered that in those with the most severe disease (stage III and stage IV cancer) who were also receiving chemotherapy, zinc supplementation was associated with a statistically improved survival rate.[109] In other words, those with the absolute worst disease, requiring the most aggressive treatment, were found to derive the greatest benefit from the antimicroinflammatory effects of zinc supplementation!

In addition to zinc's efficacy in the cancer arena, other clinical uses of the metal have reinforced its utility as an antimicroinflammatory agent.

In dermatology, acne is well established as having a significant inflammatory basis, and, in fact, the antibiotics that are used to treat it have been demonstrated not only to have antibacterial activity, but antiinflammatory effects as well.[110] Understanding this and early evidence that zinc possesses an antiinflammatory role, zinc salts were added to antibiotics in an effort to limit antibiotic resistance and enhance the efficacy of these agents in acne treatment. Indeed, the addition of zinc appeared to have an additive effect. As a result, the metal was examined as an independent treatment for acne. In one series, zinc, administered in the form of zinc gluconate, was compared to placebo in a double-blind fashion and was associated with a statistically lower inflammatory score compared to those taking placebo.[111] Further, in another study, zinc gluconate was compared to the antibiotic minocycline, and, although minocycline was superior, zinc demonstrated significant clinical benefit in the treatment of inflammatory acne.[112]

Whether examining the overt inflammation of skin diseases or the profound cellular dysfunction in cancer, it is clear that the trace element zinc has critical activity in preventing the microinflammatory cascade that affects both. Additionally, it is apparent that zinc deficiency activates the inflammatory pathways, leading to measurable differences in microinflammatory biomarkers. It is easy to focus our attention on "wonder drugs" and technological advances that have given us new treatment options, but it is also important to remember the basics and understand the critical importance that simple interventions such as trace mineral supplementation can have on our physical well-being.

VITAMINS

Vitamins represent another class of micronutrient humans require in various degrees to perform critical biological functions that involve processes such as mineral metabolism and antioxidant pathways. Theyalso serve as essential enzyme cofactors and are integrally involved with tissue development throughout our lives. Vitamins are generally classified according to their solubility in either water or fat, the importance of which relates to whether or not they can be stored or must be consumed on a regular basis. Fat-soluble vitamins, which are vitamins A, D, E, and K, can be accumulated in the body and do not require daily intake, whereas water-soluble vitamins, which include vitamin C and the eight B vitamins, are not stored, are readily excreted in the urine, and require regular intake to maintain adequate function. It has long been established that certain vitamins—vitamin C and E in particular—have potent antioxidant effects, but it has only been recognized recently that a host of vitamins have effective antimicroinflammatory properties as well.

Vitamin D

Among the vitamins with microinflammation-modulating effects, vitamin D has probably been the best studied. Vitamin D exists in two principal forms, known as vitamin D2, or ergocalciferol, and vitamin D3, also known as cholecalciferol. Vitamin D2 is primarily ingested and found abundantly in plants and mushrooms. Vitamin D3 is unique in that it is principally produced in the skin, from cholesterol, following exposure to ultraviolet B radiation. To become biologically active, vitamin D must first be converted in the liver to a molecule known as calcidiol, which is the principal circulating form of the vitamin. Calcidiol, however, is not biologically functional until it undergoes further modification in the kidney to become calcitriol. Calcitriol is critical in calcium and bone metabolism, functioning as a hormone that regulates bone turnover and coordinates with kidney, parathyroid gland, and gastrointestinal tract function. Additionally, calcitriol is vital for cellular proliferation and differentiation, and even participates in the apoptosis process. Emerging evidence has further highlighted the significance of vitamin D in microinflammatory and immune processes.[113]

In one observational series, vitamin D levels, as well as concentrations of the microinflammatory cytokine TNF-α, were examined in healthy women volunteers with varying exposures to ultraviolet B radiation. As expected, Vitamin D concentrations were statistically higher in those with regular ultraviolet B exposure compared to those without. More provocatively, there was a statistically significant inverse relationship between vitamin D levels and TNF-α concentrations, suggesting that low vitamin D activity contributes to a microinflammatory milieu, whereas normal or higher levels of vitamin D suppress such microinflammatory activity.[114]

In another investigation, serum vitamin D and CRP levels were assessed in 15,167 asymptomatic participants being followed in the National Health and Nutrition Examination Survey (NHANES). Researchers discovered that decreasing vitamin D levels were associated with a statistically significant rise in CRP concentrations, confirming another clear inverse relationship between vitamin D and microinflammatory biomarkers. Interestingly, as vitamin D levels increased above the median values for the population, CRP levels actually increased, suggesting that higher levels of vitamin D might actually be proinflammatory![115] This is another testament to the fact that more is not necessarily better, supplements cannot be taken indiscriminately, and that our physiological functions generally operate within defined parameters.

Despite studies like these demonstrating an inverse relationship between vitamin D and microinflammatory indicators, the mechanisms behind this interaction largely remained elusive until a landmark trial was published in 2012. In this investigation, the exact interplay of vitamin D's influence on microinflammatory cells was elucidated as researchers specifically examined the effect of vitamin D on the process of cytokine induction by inflammatory monocytes and macrophages. In the experiment, monocyte/macrophage production of IL-6 and TNF-α was induced by utilizing a component of bacterial cell walls known as lipopolysaccharide (LPS), which is known to strongly stimulate inflammatory cytokine release. Vitamin D treatment was found to increase the activity of a certain enzyme system that primarily functions to inhibit the release of microinflammatory cytokines produced in response to LPS stimulation.[116] As a result, the administration of a simple vitamin notably blunted a powerful stimulus for inflammatory marker release by key inflammatory cells! Not only is this commanding new information that confirms vitamin D's potent activity within the microinflammatory cascade, it illuminates the mechanism behind a previously unknown process. By identifying such functions, researchers can better define these complex pathways and derive more effective therapies to combat the microinflammation that contributes to aging and disease.

Understanding that vitamin D plays a critical role in microinflammatory pathways and that it can be used to attenuate the microinflammatory response offers promise that it may be useful as an adjunctive treatment for diseases such as cancer, which we have already established possess a significant microinflammatory component. It is interesting that epidemiologic studies in oncology have revealed a lower incidence of, and reduced mortality rates from, numerous cancers in regions with higher levels of ultraviolet B exposure.[117,118] Given the importance of ultraviolet light in the production of the physiologically active form of vitamin D, this correlation suggests that certain cancers may be vitamin D dependent. Research, in fact, has confirmed this assertion, as evidenced by the fact that circulating levels of vitamin D are inversely proportional to cancer risk![119] This association is particularly notable in colorectal cancer, where vitamin D levels and intake are inversely associated with the incidence and recurrence of colorectal adenomas, and elevated vitamin D concentrations correlate with a higher overall survival in patients with the disease.[120-122] In fact, one specific series quantified a 30% risk reduction for developing colorectal cancer in volunteers with vitamin D levels exceeding 20 nanograms/millliter (ng/ml).[123]

In addition to data regarding colorectal cancer, recent studies have demonstrated similar inverse relationships between vitamin D levels and other types of tumors. A pooled analysis of studies reporting breast cancer incidence as a function of vitamin D supplementation stratified by dose demonstrated that individuals with serum vitamin D levels of 52 ng/ml had a striking 50% reduction in risk of breast cancer compared to those with serum levels of less than 13ng/ml![124] Similarly, in a case-control study of prostate cancer risk among nineteen thousand men screened in the Helsinki Heart Study, serum levels of vitamin D greater than 20 ng/ml were associated with a 50% reduction in the risk of developing prostate cancer.[125]

These striking associations between vitamin D levels and cancer risk are certainly a provocative testament to the power of simple natural therapies in risk modification, but are there more granular data describing the mechanisms by which vitamin D can influence cancer development? Moreover, can we connect vitamin D's involvement in microinflammatory pathways to the processes that promote cancer cell formation? Indeed, current research has defined a convincing relationship between vitamin D activity, microinflammation, and tumor cell development. These mechanisms involve the all-too-familiar transcription factor NFκB, the inhibition of a class of compounds we have previously discussed known as prostaglandins, and vitamin D–dependent activity on gene expression.

Recall, the NF-κB transcription factors are intimately involved in modulating immune and microinflammatory responses and function in the final processes that stimulate the translation of messenger RNA into proteins that will become microinflammatory cytokines. Research into vitamin D activity has demonstrated that calcitriol inhibits a specific subunit of NF-κB that stimulates the production of the proinflammatory cytokine IL-8. By interfering with this particular subunit, synthesis of IL-8 dramatically decreases in the presence of vitamin D, which not only modulates the microinflammatory response, but impedes the progression of prostate cancer cell development![126] Further, NF-$\varkappa$B is implicated in prostate cancer cell resistance to radiation therapy, and vitamin D appears to counteract this action and increase the responsiveness of prostate tumors to radiation treatment.[127,128]

Another clinical link between microinflammation and prostate cancer that can potentially be modified through the anti-inflammatory effects of vitamin D involves the vitamin's apparent ability to delay the progression of a precancerous inflammatory condition of the prostate known as proliferative inflammatory atrophy (PIA). In PIA, there are microinflammatory changes within the prostate tissue that predispose to the development of cancerous cells. Multiple lines of research have demonstrated that treatment with vitamin D may potentially prevent the transformation of this precancerous tissue into overt prostate cancer.[129,130]

In addition to affecting precancerous transformation and the NF-$\varkappa$B pathways, vitamin D appears to have regulatory involvement in an important inflammatory system that involves substances we have briefly touched on known as prostaglandins. Prostaglandins are a class of fatty acid–derived compounds that are produced by most cells within the body and function in a multitude of pathways. Recall our previous discussion of the cyclooxygenase (COX) pathway and the fact that certain anti-inflammatory drugs known as COX-2 inhibitors have powerful antimicroinflammatory effects that appear chemoprotective against the formation of colorectal cancer. The COX-2 enzyme system is critical for the synthesis of prostaglandins, which, in turn, function to promote cancer cell growth as well as tumor angiogenesis. Vitamin D appears to reduce the activity of the COX-2 enzyme as well as enhance the activity of another enzyme that induces the breakdown of prostaglandins.[131] This dual effect leads to a net reduction in prostaglandin synthesis, thereby decreasing prostaglandin-induced tumor growth and angiogenesis. Interestingly, further research has indicated that vitamin D, combined with traditional nonsteroidal anti-inflammatory drugs, actually appears to inhibit prostate cancer cell growth better than vitamin D alone, suggesting that this dual attack on microinflammatory mechanisms may potentially complement current therapies for prostate cancer.[132]

A third component of vitamin D's activity in the interaction between microinflammation and cancer propagation is its ability to affect specific components of gene expression. Recall, our genes code for the formation of proteins that, in turn, perform critical functions within our bodies. Among the most important activities of genetically encoded proteins is their role as enzymes, which are essential drivers for all of our metabolic processes. Researchers have discovered that there is at least one vitaminD–responsive gene, known as MKP5, which is responsible for producing enzymes that ultimately inactivate specific stress-induced processes that lead to the liberation of microinflammatory mediators such as IL-6.[133] These insights, combined with our understanding of vitamin D's ability to regulate NF-κB activity as well as prostaglandin synthesis, provide a critical link to the microinflammatory pathways that most certainly contribute to cancer propagation. Moreover, early research in this arena provides promise for the adjunctive effect of antimicroinflammatory vitamins in cancer prevention and treatment.

By no means does this data suggest that vitamins such as cholecalciferol have the ability to prevent, cure, or independently treat cancer. However, there is compelling evidence to assert that vitamin D may be overlooked as a useful additivetherapy to traditional medicines or procedures. We must emphasize, again, that even seemingly innocuous supplements such as vitamins can have toxic effects if taken in excess, so indiscriminate usage of vitamin D or any other supplement is ill advised. When considering any nutrient additive, thorough discussions regarding appropriate dosages and costs versus benefits need to be undertaken with a health-care provider prior to utilization.

Vitamin E

Similar to vitamin D, vitamin E is a fat-soluble vitamin that appears to be significant in microinflammatory processes. Vitamin E exists in eight different forms: alpha-, beta-, gamma-, and delta-tocopherol, as well as alpha-, beta-, gamma-, and delta-tocotrienol. The most abundant form of vitamin E is gamma-tocopherol, but the most biologically active compound is alpha-tocopherol. Unlike vitamin D, vitamin E does not require any chemical conversion to its active form. Alpha-tocopherol is found in many food sources and is particularly abundant in certain vegetable oils, such as sunflower and safflower oil, wheat germ oil, olive oil, eggs, cereals, spinach, and fruits.[134]

Vitamin E deficiency is rare and usually occurs in individuals who possess fat malabsorption problems. In such individuals, severe deficiency of this fat-soluble vitamin can produce profound muscle weakness, a host of neurological disorders that can affect balance or sensation, visual disturbances, including blindness, cardiac rhythm abnormalities, and dementia.

Physiologically, Vitamin E has long been regarded as a potent antioxidant agent, but also appears to have other important functions. Vitamin E is integral in the activity of certain enzyme systems and has been found to affect gene expression. Additionally, recent investigations have demonstrated that vitamin E is involved in specific cell signaling pathways and exerts previously unrecognized antimicroinflammatory activity. Our principal focus will be vitamin E's critical involvement in redox reactions and its link to microinflammation.

From an antioxidant perspective, vitamin E's role has been well delineated for over two decades. We have previously discussed the physiological significance of different types of reactive oxygen species, including the hydroxyl and superoxide radicals. Pertinent to vitamin E's activity is an equally important reactive oxygen species known as the peroxyl radical. Whereas the superoxide radical is composed of two oxygen molecules with a net negative charge, the peroxyl radical involves an organic or carbon-centered group bound to two oxygen molecules (designated ROO, where R represents any number of carbon-based chains). Although all reactive oxygen species are important, the peroxyl radical has particular significance because it is involved in lipid peroxidation—the fundamental process in atherosclerosis that involves the oxidation of the LDL cholesterol molecule. [135]

Alpha-tocopherol potently neutralizes the peroxyl radical, thereby carrying out one of the more critical antioxidant functions in the body, as this prevents the LDL particle from being converted into a form that can be incorporated into a cholesterol plaque.[136] Even more fascinating, vitamin E actually binds to the LDL cholesterol particle such that, on average, about five to nine vitamin E molecules form a protective shield around each LDL molecule, effectively "safeguarding" the cholesterol complexfrom oxidative free radicals![137] In fact, test tube studies have shown that increasing vitamin E concentration within LDL particles actually enhances their resistance to reactive oxygen species and suppresses their uptake by macrophages, which we have previously seen is an essential step in the formation of cholesterol plaque.[138] This direct action of alpha-tocopherol at the level of the cholesterol molecule is a powerful testament to the utility of simple, natural substances in our complex metabolic systems.

In addition to vitamin E's critical activity in redox pathways, and with the LDL particle specifically, it has profound effects in the microinflammatory arena as well as other cellular processes. Multiple studies have shown that vitamin E directly reduces concentrations of microinflammatory biomarkers, including hs-CRP, TNF-α, IL-1, and other cytokines.[139-142] Moreover, alpha-tocopherol directly suppresses the production of cytokines such as IL-8, which is normally synthesized by endothelial cells, and also inhibits the adhesive activity of monocytes—another critical activity in the early phase of atherosclerosis development.[143] Additionally, vitamin E attenuates cyclooxygenase-2 (COX-2) function. This results in decreased stickiness of circulating platelets, which are critical elements in our blood that are involved in the clotting process. Intrestingly, platelets can function in both helpful and harmful ways in our bodies. On the protective side, they can clump together to essentially form a plug that stops bleeding when we get cut or sustain other trauma. On the deleterious side, they can aggregate within a heart artery, thereby stopping blood flow and producing a heart attack.[144]

Given such profound effects in many of the processes that are integral to the development and manifestation of coronary atherosclerosis, it follows that vitamin E should demonstrate clinical benefit with regard to cardiovascular end points. Although controversy has been raised due to discrepant data in studies regarding vitamin E and cardiac disease, the preponderance of information continues to support a net clinical benefit of vitamin E. In a cross-cultural European study involving thirty-nine collaborating centers in twenty-six countries, serum vitamin E levels were found to demonstrate a powerful inverse relationship with cardiac disease risk such that those with the lowest levels of alpha-tocopherol demonstrated an almost four times increased risk of cardiovascular mortality compared with those having the highest levels of the vitamin.[145]

In other series assessing the effect of long-term vitamin E supplementation as opposed to serum levels of the nutrient, similar clinical benefits were identified. These data were highlighted in a *New England Journal of Medicine* article published in 1993, where an analysis of the effect of self-reported ingestion of vitamin E was detailed in a cohort of 39,910 men followed for four years. A highly statistically significant association between the daily intake of vitamin E and the risk of developing coronary disease was identified by investigators. Specifically, those subjects in the highest quintile of vitamin E ingestion demonstrated a 40% relative risk reduction in developing coronary artery disease compared to their counterparts in the lowest quintile of alpha-tocopherol intake![146]

Whereas the prior study included only men, a similar analysis was performed among women as part of the US Nurses' Health Study. In this large prospective cohort investigation, eighty-seven thousand female nurses were enrolled with a mean follow-up period of eight years. Nurses reporting a daily intake of vitamin E of at least 100 IU (international units) experienced a 31% relative risk reduction in the combined end point of nonfatal heart attack and death from cardiovascular disease.[147] This end point is different than the previous study assessing whether or not vitamin E curtails the development of atherosclerotic disease, but is a powerful testament to the protection that it can confer against the devastating consequences of coronary disease. Considering this, it appears that the beneficial effects of alpha-tocopherol do not discriminate between the sexes.

Another investigation in the 1990s assessed the impact of vitamin E supplementation in a cohort of 11,178 patients between the ages of 67 and 105, followed in a longitudinal study known as the Established Populations for Epidemiologic Studies of the Elderly. Similar to the previous two trials, the information on vitamin supplementation was self-reported, and researchers discovered striking relative risk reductions for all-cause and cardiovascular mortality of 34% and 47%, respectively.[148] These numbers certainly mirrored results obtained in trials such as the Nurses' Health Study and the investigation by Rimm et al., but those were largely conducted in younger populations. This investigation uniquely proved that elderly patients also benefit from vitamin E supplementation and that one is never too old to derive benefits from nutrients such as alpha-tocopherol.

Looking further, researchers in the Cambridge Heart Antioxidant Study (CHAOS) assessed whether or not vitamin E supplementation would benefit those with already established atherosclerotic coronary artery disease. In this series, 2,002 patients with proven coronary disease were assigned to treatment with either 800 or 400 IU of vitamin E daily, or placebo, and were followed for a median of 510 days. As one would expect, those taking vitamin E had elevated plasma alpha-tocopherol levels compared to those ingesting placebo, with those taking 800 IU having higher concentrations than those taking 400 IU. The primary trial end point was a composite of death from any cardiac cause (heart attack, sudden cardiac arrest) andnon-fatal heart attacks. Investigators identified a statistically significant reduction in this combined outcome with the vitamin E group in both the 400 IU and 800 IU cohorts compared to placebo.[149]

In another series conducted to look at the effect of vitamin E on the progression of cholesterol plaque, researchers randomized patients to receive either 91 milligrams of vitamin E, 250 milligrams of vitamin C, a combination of the two, or placebo. The amount of plaque in the carotid arteries of the neck (a very common and easy to obtain marker of the amount of cholesterol build up present in our bodies) was quantified via ultrasound measurements before treatment and then every six months for the study duration of three years. As expected, vitamin E levels increased significantly compared to placebo in the group taking vitamin E alone or the combination pill. Similarly, vitamin C concentrations were statistically higher in the group assigned to vitamin C alone or the combination pill compared to placebo. The rate of progression of the carotid plaque was only slightly lower in the groups taking vitamin E or vitamin C alone compared to placebo, but in the combination therapy cohort, there was a robust 74%

reduction in disease progression![150] This striking effect suggests that synergistic antioxidant and antimicroinflammatory activities may exist with the combination of vitamin E and vitamin C.

There are many more trials that demonstrate similar clinical results favoring vitamin E in the population at risk for cardiovascular events, but we have iterated that some studies also demonstrate a neutral benefit of vitamin E in cardiovascular end points. It is important to assess a number of confounding issues that can occur when analyzing different research trials and weigh the potential risks and benefits of any therapy before recommending widespread adoption. At this point, it appears that vitamin E, within clinically prescribed limits, has a generally favorable profile on cardiovascular outcomes. We will continue to learn more as additional research in this arena comes to the forefront.

In addition to atherosclerotic disease, it seems that if vitamin E truly attenuates the oxidative stress and microinflammatory responses, it should demonstrate some efficacy in other clinical areas such as cancer. Indeed, many oncology trials over the years have looked at vitamin E, as well as other antioxidants and nutrients, as preventive or adjunctive therapies for cancer patients. We will examine the more salient investigations that have addressed alpha-tocopherol's role in oncology.

The first large randomized trial assessing vitamin E's efficacy in cancer prevention is known as the Chinese Cancer Prevention Study. In this series, 29,584 adults between the ages of forty and sixty-nine were randomly assigned to receive one of four nutrient combinations: (1) retinol and zinc, (2) riboflavin and niacin, (3) vitamin C and molybdenum, and (4) beta carotene, vitamin E, and selenium. The patients were followed for five years with an assessment of mortality and cancer incidence as the primary end points. The group receiving the combination of vitamin E, beta carotene, and selenium had a statistically significant reduction in mortality compared to the others, which was principally driven by decreased rates of stomach cancer and cancer overall.[151] This corroborates data in our previous discussion of the benefits of selenium and possibly demonstrates a synergy between it and vitamin E and beta carotene.

In another investigation assessing the chemopreventive properties of vitamin E, alpha-tocopherol was compared to beta carotene in male smokers. In this investigation, 29,133 male smokers between fifty and sixty-nine years of age from Finland were randomly assigned to receive either alpha-tocopherol alone, beta carotene alone, both beta carotene and alpha-tocopherol in combination, or placebo. The follow-up period was five to eight years, and the primary end point was actually an assessment of the two vitamins' effect on lung cancer. Interestingly, neither beta carotene nor alpha-tocopherol demonstrated any chemoprotective effect against lung cancer. However, alpha-tocopherol did appear to be associated with a reduced incidence of both prostate and colorectal cancer.[152] At the time this trial was conducted, this observation was unique, but subsequent trials have produced similar findings.[153,154]

Cancer mortality was an additional end point in the Established Populations for Epidemiologic Studies of the Elderly investigation discussed previously. Although not as robust as the reductions in all-cause and cardiovascular mortality, this study, in an aged population, demonstrated a respectable 23% relative risk reduction in cancer mortality for the 11,178 patient cohort.[148] In the paper, cancers were not stratified by anatomic location, but this reduction certainly provides compelling evidence for the chemopreventive effects of vitamin E.

Similar to those in cardiovascular disease trials, outcomes with vitamin E supplementation have met with controversy in the cancer arena. Based upon the discrepant results, no cancer society is willing to recommend the widespread use of vitamin E for chemoprevention, but additional trials are being conducted to better resolve the incongruity between different investigations. Nonetheless, the benefit of vitamin E supplementation, similar to many other nutrients and even prescription medications, needs to be assessed on an individual basis with collaboration between patients and their health-care providers.

PLANT-DERIVED POLYPHENOLS

Plant-derived polyphenols are a class of compounds that share common chemical structural rings known as phenol groups. Polyphenols are also referred to as flavonoids or flavonols (although in chemical terms, these are actually different substances) and in nature are abundant in plant leaves, where they serve as antioxidants. Some polyphenols known as phytoalexins are produced by plants in response to infection and protect them against invading organisms such as fungus or bacteria. A host of dietary plants contain polyphenols, but they are most commonly found in fruits, vegetables, legumes, grains, tea, and wine. The polyphenols most extensively studied in the microinflammation, antioxidant, and antiaging arenas are resveratrol, curcumin, and quercetin.[155] We will examine each of these agents and discuss their utility in preventing disease and the aging process.

Resveratrol

Resveratrol is perhaps the best known of the polyphenols and has certainly had the lion's share of press over the years as it gained the reputation of being the key substance in red wine that is responsible for its health benefits. The "French paradox," initially detailed in 1992 by Dr. Serge Renaud and colleagues, centered on red wine as the component of the French diet that explained why French people, despite having a diet high in saturated fats and a greater than normal utilization of cigarettes, had a statistically lower mortality rate from cardiac disease.[156] Although some of the health benefits of wine seem to be related to the alcohol component itself, studies have demonstrated that resveratrol seems to be the most biologically active ingredient with regard to antioxidant, anti-inflammatory, antiaging and anticancer effects. We will explore these in detail.

Although we have focused on wine's resveratrol content, it is noteworthy that this polyphenol is actually found in over seventy plant species. Resveratrol is a phytoalexin, which, as we previously described, means that it protects its host plant from fungal, viral, and bacterial attack, as well as ultraviolet radiation and ozone.[157] One of the principal reasons resveratrol is synonymous with red wine is that the grapes used to make these generally contain maximum concentrations of the polyphenol. In fact, the average concentration of resveratrol in red wine is anywhere from one and a half to a hundred times greater than that in white wines, depending on the specific varietal that is used.[158]

As an antioxidant, resveratrol has been shown to inhibit the production of reactive oxygen species by inflammatory cells. In a study conducted at Barcelona University in Spain, researchers utilized an inflammatory stimulus we have discussed before, lipopolysaccharide (LPS), to induce macrophages to produce their principal reactive oxygen species—superoxide and hydrogen peroxide. In the Barcelona protocol, LPS stimulation of macrophages was performed with and without resveratrol administration, and reactive oxygen species concentrations were quantified under both conditions. Resveratrol administration resulted in a significant decrease in both superoxide and hydrogen peroxide production compared to controls not receiving the agent. Moreover, resveratrol was noted to markedly inhibit the LPS induction of the cyclooxygenase-2 enzyme system, resulting in a significant decrease in the production of prostaglandins.[159] Based upon this, and other trials, it is undeniable that resveratrol exerts powerful antioxidant effects.

Regarding microinflammation attenuation, studies with resveratrol have identified a variety of mechanisms through which the polyphenol acts. In one series, resveratrol was administered following an LPS stimulus designed to induce an inflammatory response in lung tissue. A dose-related inhibition in the number of inflammatory white blood cells was noted in the lung tissue of resveratrol-treated subjects compared to those who received LPS stimulation alone. Additionally, the expression of a host of microinflammatory biomarkers was significantly attenuated in the resveratrol group, particularly TNF-α and IL-1β. Interestingly, this occurred without inhibition of NF-ᴋB action, which we have seen at the center of activity in a multitude of other antimicroinflammatory substances.[160]

Despite these results, other research has demonstrated that resveratrol actually exerts some antimicroinflammatory activity through inhibition of the NF-ᴋB transcription factor. In one investigation that examined resveratrol's effect in multiple cell lines, the polyphenol was shown to directly block the tumor necrosis factor- induced activation of NF-ᴋB in a dose-dependent manner.[161] In another series involving liver cancer cells, resveratrol was found to inhibit NF-ᴋB expression, which, in turn, reduced the TNF-α-mediated activity of a specific group of enzymes known as matrix metalloproteinases. These enzymes are also elevated in inflammatory states and can be used in studies as surrogate markers of microinflammation.[162] Finally, in an investigation involving microinflammatory activity in adipocytes, resveratrol was found to inhibit the DNA binding activity of NF-ᴋB under TNF-α stimulation, resulting in suppression of the transcription and secretion of monocyte chemoattractant protein (MCP-1), which, as we have previously seen, is responsible for macrophage infiltration into fatty tissue.[163] Despite results in the previous study that demonstrated no NF-ᴋB inhibition with resveratrol, it appears that other lines of evidence suggest that resveratrol indeed affects the action of this important transcription factor. This likely illustrates that resveratrol affects microinflammatory processes in different ways, some related to NF-κB activity, and others not.

Considering alternative mechanisms, research has established that resveratrol exerts antimicroinflammatory activity through inhibition of the cyclooxygenase (COX) pathways. Different investigations, however, have revealed variable effects of resveratrol on the COX-1 and COX-2 systems. In an analysis of COX induction in liver and lung tissue, investigators determined that the polyphenol strongly inhibits COX-1 activity.[164] Similarly, in a study designed specifically to assess the differential effects of resveratrol on the COX enzymes, joint research from the United States and Italy demonstrated strong inhibition of the COX-1 enzyme by resveratrol, but negligible effect on COX-2.[165] As noted previously, resveratrol has also been shown to inhibit the LPS-mediated expression of COX-2, thereby decreasing levels of microinflammatory prostaglandins.[150] In yet another series, resveratrol was shown to reduce colon tissue injury, white blood cell infiltration, and concentrations of a specific prostaglandin known as PGD2 as a function of COX-2 inhibition without COX-1 involvement.[166] Based upon these studies, it appears that resveratrol inhibits both COX-1 and COX-2 pathways, producing reductions in microinflammatory prostaglandins in either case. Further research will be needed to determine under which circumstances resveratrol will affect COX-1 versus COX-2 enzymes and which of these inhibitory functions will be most critical in suppressing microinflammation.

Clinically, the anti-inflammatory activity of resveratrol has probably been best explored in the respiratory disease arena. Both asthma and emphysema are known to have a large inflammatory component, and evidence that antioxidant and antimicroinflammatory activity could attenuate these disease processes was initially discovered in epidemiological studies. In the prospective Nurses' Health Study of over seventy-two thousand women, the risk of chronic obstructive pulmonary disease (COPD), or emphysema, was assessed in a cohort followed between 1984 and 2000. In individuals consuming a largely "Western" diet, consisting of processed foods with high fat content and minimal antioxidants, the risk of developing COPD was 31% higher compared to individuals consuming a diet rich in fruits, vegetables, and whole grains.[167]

The Nurses' Health Study failed to demonstrate an increased risk of asthma associated with the Western diet, but another series conducted as part of the International Study of Asthma and Allergies in Childhood (ISAAC) did reveal such a correlation. In ISAAC, a cross-sectional cohort study of 1,321 children was conducted to ascertain the relationship between asthma and dietary patterns. Children consuming a higher fat, lower antioxidant diet compared to those ingesting decreased quantities of fattier foods demonstrated a significant increase in asthma symptoms and an abnormal response to a test known as bronchial hyperresponsiveness—a surrogate for diagnosing exercise-induced, or provokable, asthma.[168]

Beyond these large epidemiological series that suggest a correlation between low-antioxidant diets and inflammatory lung diseases, several other investigations have demonstrated that the consumption of foods rich in antioxidants such as resveratrol are associated with improved outcomes for these conditions. In a case-control study involving 1,471 patients aged sixteen to fifty years conducted in Europe, the association between asthma and dietary antioxidants in fruits, vegetables, and red wine were assessed. There was a strongly negative correlation between asthma development and individuals in the highest quintiles of apple consumption, which consisted of greater than five apples per week. Although not as strong, a negative correlation was also found between the highest quintiles of onion, tea, and red wine consumption, with the study overall suggesting a decrease in asthma severity in individuals consuming the highest levels of antioxidant-rich food and drinks, particularly apples.[169] Obviously, these foods contain many antioxidants besides resveratrol, but the red wine correlation certainly corroborates resveratrol's potent antimicroinflammatory properties.

With regard to resveratrol's activity in other diseases, there is robust evidence to suggest that this important polyphenol has the potential to attenuate processes that contribute to atherosclerosis, cancer, and even aging. We have already discussed how endothelial dysfunction is paramount to the development of clinically significant atherosclerotic disease, and that impaired function of endothelial cells leads to untoward effects such as blood vessel constriction. The net result of blood vessel constriction or blood vessel dilatation is mediated through the opposing forces of a vasodilator we have discussed known as nitric oxide and a vasoconstrictor known as endothelin-1 (ET-1). In states of endothelial dysfunction, nitric oxide production by endothelial cells is decreased, and their release of ET-1 is enhanced. Studies have revealed that resveratrol exerts a dual effect on these vasoactive substances by preventing the production and release of ET-1 by inhibiting its gene expression and enhancing the activity of nitric oxide.[170] More importantly, compelling research has revealed that in subjects with baseline endothelial dysfunction, resveratrol supplementation, as well as red wine consumption, results in restoration of endothelial function with concomitant reduction in ET-1 levels.[171] It is amazing to realize that a simple plant-derived substance has the power to alter physiological processes at the genetic level and translate these modifications into potentially beneficial cardioprotective effects.

We have discussed resveratrol's effect on the COX enzyme systems and its importance in attenuating the microinflammatory response. Moreover, we have discussed the critical role that microinflammation plays in all stages of atherosclerosis, from initiation through plaque rupture. Resveratrol's ability to inhibit COX-1 and COX-2 activity leads to vital reductions in prostaglandins that not only function to propagate the microinflammatory response, but are also involved in the process of platelet aggregation that occurs when atherosclerotic plaques rupture.[164,165] As a result, resveratrol has the potential to serve as a critical barrier in the entire atherosclerotic process, tempering the microinflammatory milieu that exists from initiation through propagation and ultimately rupture of an atherosclerotic plaque, as well as reducing prostaglandins that induce the formation of platelet-rich clot that ensues following plaque rupture.

In addition to mitigating the harmful effects of the cyclooxygenase pathways, resveratrol has the potential to modulate another important process in the atherosclerosis cascade—lipid peroxidation. Recall, one of the critical steps in plaque formation is the oxidative modification of the LDL molecule that transforms it into a particle that is readily taken up by monocytes and macrophages. Resveratrol has been shown in multiple series to inhibit the deleterious oxidation of LDL particles, rendering them unsuitable for uptake by such inflammatory cells.[172-174] This powerful inhibition occurs at a critical juncture in the atherosclerotic process, highlighting the importance of polyphenols in the protection against the premature development of lethal cardiac disease.

Another beneficial cardiovascular effect that resveratrol can exert involves platelet physiology. Recall that one of the fundamental processes occurring during a heart attack is the aggregation, or sticking together, of platelets after an atherosclerotic plaque has ruptured. Normally, drugs such as aspirin are used to decrease platelet stickiness, but several studies have demonstrated that resveratrol also possesses the ability to hinder platelet activity at multiple critical points. The first step in platelet activation involves the adhesion of these circulating blood elements to the substance known as collagen, which becomes exposed when the endothelium is injured. Collagen is a protein that is used for structural support throughout the body and is abundant in tissues such as blood vessels, tendons, ligaments, skin, cartilage and bone. When the collagen from blood vessels is exposed during endothelial injury, resveratrol has been shown to not only decrease platelet adhesion to this important structural protein,, but also decrease the expression of collagen mRNA![175,176] Additional investigation has revealed that a second mechanism through which resveratrol impedes platelet activation is via the inhibition of calcium influx into stimulated platelets, which is an important step in increasing platelet aggregability, or their propensity to clump together.[177] Lastly, resveratrol has been shown to decrease the endothelial cell and monocyte production of a protein known as tissue factor, which is a component of the clotting cascade that becomes activated when atherosclerotic plaques rupture.[178,179] Through three powerful and independent mechanisms, this seemingly simple compound can block one of the key processes that leads to arterial blockage and potential fatal heart attacks.

A final cardioprotective property of resveratrol involves its ability to constrain smooth muscle cell proliferation. Smooth muscle cells are found in the walls of arteries and principally function to allow the blood vessels to expand and contract under the appropriate conditions. Unlike the muscles we use to perform voluntary, everyday functions like walking, picking up objects or writing, smooth muscles are under involuntary control, reacting to instructions from the nervous system or local chemical signals. In addition to their role in maintaining the appropriate amount of contraction or relaxation of blood vessels, smooth muscle cells have an important function in the proliferative phase of plaque formation. . Specifically, smooth muscle cell migration and development is integral to the progression of the atherosclerotic plaque, and these cells are capable of accumulating oxidized lipids, similar to macrophages and monocytes. Research has shown that resveratrol has the ability to block the proliferation of smooth muscle cells within the walls of arteries, thereby inhibiting one of the steps that leads to atherosclerotic plaque propagation.[180,181] Combining all of these properties, it appears that there is a strong physiological basis for the French paradox, and plant-derived polyphenols are an important natural defense against microinflammation-induced cardiovascular disease progression.

In addition to its activity in coronary disease, exciting research has revealed resveratrol's potential to attenuate cancer. As we have seen, the process of carcinogenesis is quite complex and involves multiple steps that ultimately converge to induce uncontrolled cellular growth. Resveratrol appears to exert anticancer effects through various mechanisms including inhibiting proliferation and angiogenesis and promoting apoptosis. Moreover, the polyphenol seems to demonstrate chemopreventive activity as well. We shall explore each of these facets in more detail.

From a chemoprevention standpoint, we have discussed the importance of the COX system, particularly as it relates to colorectal cancer. Moreover, we have described the inhibitory effects of resveratrol on the COX enzymes. As a result, it should not be difficult to extrapolate an antitumor effect of resveratrol mediated through the same COX system. Indeed, studies have demonstrated that resveratrol not only suppresses the expression of the COX-2 gene, but directly inhibits the activity of the COX-2 enzyme system.[164,165] Further, through its antioxidant properties, resveratrol has the potential to disrupt the initiation of cancer cell transformation by inhibiting the activation of procarcinogenic molecules that, if left unchecked, could bind to DNA and produce genetic mutations.[173] Resveratrol's powerful combination of antioxidant and antimicroinflammatory activity—two processes at the heart of tumor development—is an amazing dual action in the ever-growing arena of cancer prevention.

In addition to these compelling pharmacopreventive properties, resveratrol can impede cancer development by promoting apoptosis. Older studies revealed that resveratrol induced specific protein-mediated signals on leukemia cells that triggered the apoptotic cascade.[182] Additionally, resveratrol was determined to induce apoptosis in epidermal, lymphoblast, and fibroblast cell lines by activating the p53 gene, which, as we discussed previously, codes for the tumor suppressor p53 protein that is integral to the apoptotic process.[183] This is akin to resveratrol throwing the proverbial wrench into a machine that causes the gears to jam, ultimately resulting in the destruction of the machine. Through these mechanisms, resveratrol appears to directly induce the cellular death that is crucial to preventing tumor cell propagation. It is astounding to realize that such a profound effect can come from a simple natural compound.

We have seen that one of the fundamental processes in cancer promotion is the uncontrolled growth, or proliferation, of cells that form the enlarging tumor. In addition to its other effects, resveratrol appears to have the capacity to inhibit this proliferative response. In concentrations mirroring that found in wine, resveratrol has demonstrated the ability to stunt the propagation of several cell types in a time- and concentration-dependent fashion.[184,185] In a study examining human breast cancer cell lines, resveratrol was found to suppress cell growth in all types and also antagonized the effect of a known, potent cancer cell stimulator![186] Part of this appears related to the p53 activity described previously, but, rather than always stimulating programmed cell death, resveratrol seems to also trigger a state of arrested development within certain cells, thus halting their proliferative activity. It matters little whether the cell is programmed to die or simply is given a signal to stop multiplying—the ultimate result is its inability to proliferate and create an enlarging cancerous mass.

We have previously addressed the importance of angiogenesis, or the development of new blood vessels, for tumor growth and metastasis. One of the most important factors involved in the angiogenesis process is known as vascular endothelial growth factor (VEGF), which functions much like fertilizer to promote new blood vessels to form. Studies have shown that resveratrol inhibits VEGF in several different ways, thereby shutting down the stimulus for tumor cells to form new vessels. In multiple myeloma cell lines, resveratrol has been shown to inhibit the genetic expression and secretion of VEGF.[187] Similarly, in a study of breast cancer cells, resveratrol, at high doses, was found to decrease the secretion of VEGF in both test tube and animal subjects.[188] Decreasing the ability of tumor cells to develop new blood vessels is a critical step in impeding the growth of cancer cells, and these, as well as other studies, continue to demonstrate the commanding potential of resveratrol as an anticancer agent.

Clinically, the mechanisms above have translated to observable therapeutic benefits of resveratrol in the cancer management arena, particularly as an adjunct to conventional therapies. In one series, the regulatory effect of resveratrol was examined relative to the inhibitory potential of a vitamin D analog. Prior research has revealed that a specific form of vitamin D known as vitamin D_3 inhibits growth of breast cancer cells, which gives it the potential to sensitize breast cancer cells to standard treatments. This is much like weakening an opponent in a boxing match by subjecting him to heavy exertion immediately prior to the fight. The weakened, or sensitized, breast cancer cells, similar to the fighter, are more vulnerable to attack once they have been exposed to vitamin D_3. In this investigation, researchers found that resveratrol enhanced vitamin D_3's sensitizing ability, further augmenting the growth-inhibiting effects of the vitamin on breast cancer cells and improving the activity of a standard breast cancer drug known as tamoxifen![189] As a result, the combination of resveratrol and vitamin D_3 appears to pack a one-two punch that weakens breast cancer cells and makes them more susceptible to treatment with a standard anticancer therapy such as tamoxifen.

In addition to breast cancer, resveratrol appears to be active in sensitizing other tumor cells to standard treatments or overtly preventing their growth and proliferation. In two studies, specific drug-refractory lymphoma cells were pretreated with resveratrol and then subjected to standard chemotherapy regimens. The resveratrol-treated cells actually demonstrated improved response to several drugs, confirming the polyphenol's ability to sensitize the cancer cells to standard treatments.[190] In isolated human leukemia cells, exposure to resveratrol produced a potent apoptotic response, resulting in a significant reduction in leukemia cells.[191] Similarly, in an investigation of thyroid cancer cell lines, resveratrol produced a statistically significant reduction in tumor cell proliferation.[192] Finally, in an examination of prostate cancer, resveratrol treatment resulted in decreased cell growth through apoptosis and diminished the levels of prostate-specific antigen (PSA)—a common tumor marker used in the detection and monitoring of prostate cancer.[193,194] These potent effects pave the path for potentially new synergistic therapies that can combine the power of natural agents, such as resveratrol, with traditional medicines to create a more effective response.

Perhaps one of the more provocative areas of resveratrol research involves its potential to retard the aging process. As we have seen, senescence is a complex, multifaceted interplay between a host of metabolic and physiological actions. Although we are still somewhat in the Dark Ages of our understanding of what happens as we grow older, we know that the aging process is marked by increased oxidative stress and that reactive oxygen species are implicated in age-related derangements at the cellular level. Moreover, we have seen that microinflammation is intimately tied to the process of cellular senescence. Given resveratrol's established efficacy as a potent antioxidant and antimicroinflammatory agent, it should come as no surprise that this polyphenol has received considerable attention as an antiaging compound. We have extensively reviewed resveratrol's effectiveness in microinflammation and oxidative cellular processes and will now examine resveratrol's other mechanisms in the antiaging arena.

One of the more recent breakthroughs in understanding the cellular senescence process has been the identification of an enzyme known as sirtuin 1 (SIRT1). Interestingly, SIRT1 is the human counterpart of an enzyme in yeast known as silent information regulator 2 protein (Sir2p). Early studies demonstrated that increased activity of the gene coding for Sir2p actually improved the longevity of yeast, providing an enzyme-related connection to the antiaging process.[195] We previously discussed that caloric restriction is the only dietary modification that correlates with life span extension across multiple species, and follow-up research in the Sir2p arena determined that caloric restriction could not improve the longevity in yeast with defective genes coding for the enzyme.[196] Researchers have concluded that this is prima facie evidence that Sir2p and its human counterpart, SIRT1, are responsible for mediating the antiaging and health-promoting effects of caloric restriction!

With this exciting revelation, researchers next investigated substances that could stimulate the SIRT1 enzyme. Among the different compounds tested, resveratrol proved to be the most effective and significantly increased the activity of Sir2p and SIRT1. Moreover, when resveratrol was administered to the yeast, they demonstrated a profound increase in both maximum and average life span![197] Expanding this work to higher-level organisms, resveratrol has demonstrated analogous antiaging effects in flies, worms, fish, and mice![198-201] Humans are obviously a far cry from mice and other lower life forms, but all great human discoveries generally have foundations in animal research, providing us with an optimistic outlook on resveratrol. Moreover, the fact that the SIRT1 enzyme system seems to perform the same activity across species lines provides encouragement that the end results of activating this system will translate into similar effects in higher-level organisms.

A more recent study in human subjects has provided some additional provocative evidence for resveratrol in the antiaging and metabolic health space. In this investigation, which was conducted in the Netherlands, resveratrol was administered to obese men in a randomized double-blind fashion for thirty days with the goal of assessing its effects on a host of metabolic parameters. Researchers discovered that resveratrol-treated subjects had increased SIRT1 activity, similar to the findings in lower organisms detailed previously. Moreover, those receiving resveratrol demonstrated statistically significant reductions in systolic blood pressure, insulin, and glucose, and also showed enhanced insulin sensitivity compared to the placebo group.[202] Given the importance of insulin activity in the antimicroinflammatory and aging processes that we have already described, it is compelling to understand that resveratrol significantly impacts this physiology. Moreover, the confirmation of enhanced SIRT1 activity validates that which we have seen in lower organisms and provides convincing evidence that resveratrol may exert a positive impact on adverse processes that are associated with the aging process. Admittedly, this is a far cry from stating that resveratrol is the fountain of youth, but the data available thus far suggests that this plant-derived agent my prove to be an important part of maintaining healthy metabolic function as we age.

Curcumin

Curcumin is the major polyphenol constituent in the spice commonly known as turmeric, and is principally responsible for its characteristic brilliant yellow color, but, more importantly, its health benefits. Turmeric is a member of the ginger family, is derived from the roots and stems of the *Curcuma longa* plant, is harvested largely in India and other regions in Southeast Asia, and has long been used in Ayurvedic medicine as a treatment for inflammatory conditions. Curcumin, as the principally active component of the spice, has been extensively studied and seems to possess potent antioxidant, antimicroinflammatory, and antimicrobial activity.[203] We shall explore curcumin's mechanism of action in detail and examine its efficacy in the antimicroinflammatory and disease management arenas.

Curcumin's antioxidant activity has been well cited in medical and lay literature for decades. This property of curcumin has largely been investigated in laboratory animals, but, as we shall see, newer research in human models has shown promising results. In one investigation, utilizing a rat model of oxidative stress related to lead toxicity, curcumin was found to produce a decrease in lipid peroxidation, as well as an increase in the activity of the antioxidant enzymes superoxide dismutase and catalase.[204] Similarly, in another rat model, curcumin supplementation was found to increase the activity of a naturally produced antioxidant known as glutathione peroxidase by 21%.[205] In a study of human blood cells exposed to a known oxidant called methylglyoxal, curcumin administration was found to reduce reactive oxygen species production, decrease markers of oxidative stress, diminish DNA damage, and inhibit methylglyoxal-induced apoptosis.[206] More provocatively, however, a recent study from investigators at Ohio State University, presented at the 2012 Experimental Biology meeting in San Diego, demonstrated that administration of a more absorbable preparation of curcumin to healthy human subjects produced an increase in the endogenous antioxidant catalase![207] This compelling new information suggests that the foundational research in animals and human cell lines translates to a quantifiable antioxidant effect in healthy human subjects and corroborates one of the historical properties of this potent polyphenol.

Translating this antioxidant activity into a more clinically relevant example, curcumin appears to exert potentially beneficial effects on the LDL cholesterol molecule. As we have discussed, an important step in the atherosclerotic process is the oxidation of LDL particles, which make them "attractive" for uptake by macrophages and monocytes. A study conducted at the University of Illinois assessed curcumin's ability to impede this oxidation process, thereby making the LDL cholesterol less likely to be incorporated into an atherosclerotic plaque. Utilizing human endothelial cells and standard laboratory models for oxidizing LDL molecules, researchers discovered that low concentrations of curcumin were able to prevent the LDL oxidation process.[208] By thwarting this critical step in the atherosclerotic process, curcumin demonstrates promise as a novel therapeutic agent in the fight against cholesterol plaque formation in arteries.

From a microinflammation standpoint, curcumin seems to modulate many familiar pathways. Research has clearly demonstrated that curcumin suppresses the activation of NF-κB, which, as we have seen, is an integral component of microinflammatory pathways and is expressed in most cancer types. This NF-κB suppression has been observed in a wide variety of experimental models, including tumors grown in laboratory mice, as well as human patients, with pancreatic cancer and multiple myeloma.[209,210] Looking further downstream in the microinflammatory process, inhibiting NF-κB results in the downregulation of both COX-2 and nitric oxide synthase enzyme systems as well as a decrease in the production of critical cytokines such as TNF-α, IL-1, IL-2, IL-6, IL-8, and IL-12.[211,212] Recall that nitric oxide synthase is the enzyme responsible for catalyzing the production of nitric oxide, which, in turn, regulates vascular tone and is involved in angiogenesis. By shutting down the expression of both the COX-2 and nitric oxide synthase enzyme systems and diminishing the release of cytokines via this NF-κB suppression, curcumin can play a critical role in hindering important microinflammatory processes and preventing tumor cell proliferation and spread.

Similar to resveratrol, curcumin appears to inhibit the expression of vascular endothelial growth factor (VEGF). Recall, VEGF functions as the "fertilizer" for angiogenesis, which is a critical process for the growth and metastasis of tumor cells. One study has demonstrated that curcumin actually enhances the antitumor properties of a chemotherapy agent called gemcitabine in subjects with pancreatic cancer, specifically with regard to VEGF inhibition and the resultant decrease in angiogenesis.[213] Similarly, in a study of ovarian cancer, curcumin was found to produce a potent reduction in angiogenesis, thereby inhibiting the growth of these cancer cells as well.[214] By choking off a tumor's blood supply by suppressing its ability to form new blood vessels, curcumin inhibits vital nutrients from feeding the growing cancer. Through this activity, this powerful plant-derived substance may prove to be a potent adjunct to standard cancer therapy.

In addition to its activity with VEGF, curcumin offers promise in attenuating cancer formation and propagation through other mechanisms. In a study of human colon cancer cells, researchers from the University of Texas Medical Branch at Galveston utilized a tumor-inducer known as neurotensin to stimulate interleukin-8 (IL-8) expression and release, which, in turn, is known to promote cancer progression. Subsequently, curcumin was administered and discovered to block the neurotensin-mediated liberation of IL-8 and its subsequent effect on cancer cell migration![215] This is an eloquent example of the interplay between the microinflammatory process and cancer promotion, with the inflammatory cytokine IL-8 being the direct instigator that is readily inhibited by the potent antimicroinflammatory effects of curcumin.

In a study involving human breast cancer cell lines, curcumin's efficacy in suppressing COX-2, VEGF, and NF-$\varkappa$B was examined, with a secondary goal of delineating the resultant effect of this inhibition on metastatic disease. Curcumin administration clearly produced marked decreases in the expression of VEGF, COX-2, and NF-$\varkappa$B, the combination of which would be expected to induce impaired tumor proliferation and spread. Indeed, the subjects receiving curcumin supplementation demonstrated profound reductions in the incidence of breast cancer metastasis to the lungs![216] This has provided yet another potent example of curcumin's effect on critical microinflammatory pathways and its ability to attenuate cancer growth and spread.

Beyond examining curcumin's effect on surrogates of microinflammatory activity, its clinical action has been investigated in a multitude of studies utilizing patients under active cancer treatment regimens. As we have previously seen, there has been strong interest in substances that have activity against COX-2, particularly in the arena of colorectal cancer and precancerous colorectal adenomas, making curcumin an ideal investigational agent in these populations. One series assessed the efficacy of curcumin combined with another polyphenol agent, quercetin, in patients with familial adenomatous polyposis (FAP) who had previously undergone colon removal for extensive polyp disease. Patients were treated with the combination for a mean of six months and demonstrated no appreciable toxicity. At the end of the study, follow-up colonoscopy revealed a mean decrease of 60% in the number of polyps as well as a 51% decrease in polyp size.[217] This promising data has led to the development of several more research protocols that will further investigate the provocative chemopreventive properties of polyphenols and other natural agents in colorectal cancer.

In another study involving patients with premalignant and early invasive lesions of the colon and rectum, curcumin was administered in an escalating dose fashion for three months. Tissue examination revealed improvement in 28% of the subjects without significant toxicity at the highest doses of curcumin.[218] This study corroborated the previous safety profile of curcumin at high doses, but obviously gives promise to its potential in attenuating the progression of early colorectal cancer.

Regarding the aging process, it is important to reiterate that senescence itself is difficult to define and is not the result of a single pathway in all individuals. We do understand that senescence seems to involve the interplay between chronic oxidative stress and low-level inflammation that results in damage to DNA and other cellular constituents. Given the complexities of the aging process, no universal definition of aging has truly emerged, making research into aging more problematic from the perspective of defining appropriate study end points. . To date, no major trial has been conducted to assess curcumin's efficacy in this arena, but scientists certainly speculate that curcumin has all of the properties that would prevent cellular senescence, as we have seen that it is a potent antioxidant and antimicroinflammatory agent. As the process of cellular senescence is better understood, we hope to better define research outcomes so that we can formally assess the activity of agents such as curcumin against these parameters.

Quercetin

Quercetin is another of the plant-derived polyphenols that is abundant in a variety of fruits, vegetables, and other food sources. Some of the highest concentrations of quercetin are leaf-derived and found in black and green tea as well as lovage. Capers are another potent source of the polyphenol, with concentrations of quercetin approximating that found in tea and lovage. Lower, but still abundant, amounts of quercetin are found in onions, apples, red grapes, and citrus fruits. Additionally, other sources of this polyphenol include parsley, tomatoes, broccoli, raspberries, and cranberries. Given its presence in red grapes, quercetin is another constituent of red wine that is believed to impart some of its myriad health benefits.[219,220]

As an antimicroinflammatory agent, quercetin has been well studied and appears to exert its inhibitory effect on inflammatory pathways via multiple mechanisms. In a study dating back to the early 1980s, quercetin was discovered to inhibit the enzyme phospholipase A_2 (PLA_2), which is responsible for releasing arachidonic acid from cell membranes.[221] Recall, arachidonic acid is a fatty acid that has critical inflammatory activity, as it is a precursor to substances such as prostaglandins that are directly involved in the microinflammatory response. By inhibiting the release of this fatty acid from the membranes of cells and thereby reducing downstream substrates necessary for promoting the microinflammatory cascade, quercetin is able to effectively attenuate the microinflammatory state at a very early stage.

In addition to its activity on PLA_2, quercetin demonstrates inhibitory action on the familiar COX system. In particular, studies have demonstrated that quercetin demonstrates potent inhibition of the COX-1 system, which, as we have briefly mentioned before, is responsible for producing prostaglandins and thromboxanes from arachidonic acid. Further, quercetin appears to demonstrate at least moderate inhibition of COX-2.[221] Obviously, the combined effect of COX-1 and COX-2 inhibition is a profound reduction in prostaglandin synthesis, which, when combined with quercetin's effect on PLA_2, has the potential to significantly reduce the microinflammatory milieu.

By inhibiting microinflammatory pathways as just described, we have previously seen that biomarkers of inflammation are expected to be reduced. Studies have confirmed that quercetin administration is indeed associated with significant reductions of microinflammatory biomarkers, particularly IL-1β, IL-6, and TNF-α.[222,223] At this point, it should come as no surprise that this is mediated through suppression of the NF-κB system, which we have seen is a critical component of microinflammatory pathways throughout the body.

Quercetin is probably one of the best studied of the polyphenols, and the molecular mechanisms leading to its effects in the microinflammatory arena have been meticulously detailed. Before discussing these mechanisms, however, it will be helpful to describe what is known as the cell cycle, cell replication cycle, or cell division cycle to better understand where quercetin exerts its effects.

The cell cycle refers to the process by which cells divide so that they can duplicate and proliferate—a progression that is necessary for both normal cells as well as cancers. The cell cycle is divided into four distinct stages termed: G_1 phase, S phase, G_2 phase and M phase (see figure 1). The G_1 phase, S phase, and G_2 phases combined are often termed "interphase" and represent the preparatory stages for cell division, which occurs in the M phase. The first stage of the cell cycle, G_1, is generally considered the growth period and involves a high rate of amino acid synthesis, which will be used as the building blocks for the construction of proteins and enzymes necessary for DNA construction. The G_1 phase is variable in length, but begins at the end of the previous M phase (which is detailed below) and continues until the initiation of DNA synthesis. At the end of the G_1 phase, the first cell cycle "checkpoint" is encountered, where certain "credentials" must be present in order for the cell to progress further. These cell cycle checkpoints function much like sentries in a guardhouse, limiting the passage of cells from one phase to the next if they possess intrinsic defects. At the G_1 checkpoint, two protein complexes, named CDK4/6-cyclin D and CDK2-cyclin E, are the guardhouse custodians and determine whether or not the cell has the qualifications to move forward to the next phase. If a cell is deemed faulty at this juncture, its further development will be arrested, and it will be prohibited from completing the cell cycle. Most other cells will progress to the next stage. However, some normal tissue constituents, such as liver cells, will enter a resting phase where they do not proceed any further.

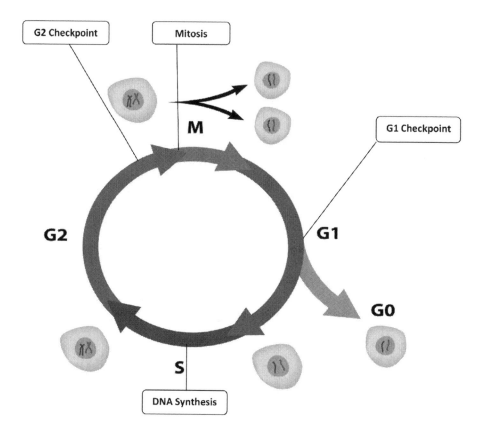

Figure 1: The Cell Cycle G_1 marks the beginning of the cell cycle where rapid growth and protein synthesis ensues. At the G_1 checkpoint, defective cells are arrested from proceeding any further. Those that continue forth move into the S phase, where DNA synthesis occurs. This is followed by another growth phase, G_2, where additional proteins and constituents needed to complete cell division are manufactured. Another checkpoint occurs at the end of G_2, and if the cell is qualified, it moves into the final phase, M, where mitosis occurs, leading to the production of two daughter cells from the original cell.

Cells that fulfill criteria for successful passage beyond the G_1 stage then enter the S phase, which marks the beginning of DNA synthesis. The S phase occurs very quickly, as this is the stage during which the DNA molecule is naked and vulnerable. Within the S phase, components of DNA are most susceptible to damage by external factors such as reactive oxygen species, drugs, or other damaging substances, so the cellular machinery attempts to complete the synthesis of the DNA molecule quickly to avert any untoward effects. During the S phase, all of the chromosomes are replicated, thereby creating a duplicate set of the entire DNA sequence within the cell. Once this matching DNA set has been entirely duplicated, the S phase is complete.

Next is the G_2 phase, which, similar to G_1, involves a high rate of protein synthesis. Additionally, cells during G_2 phase produce cylindrical structures known as microtubules that, as we shall see, are necessary to complete the process of mitosis in the M phase. During G_2, the cell grows significantly as it prepares to split into two identical daughter cells. At the end of the G_2 phase, the cell reaches what is known as the G_2 checkpoint, where a specific substance known as mitosis-promoting factor or maturation-promiting factor (MPF) must be activated in order for the cell to continue on. If MPF is present and functionally active, the cell will continue on to the M phase. If MPF is absent, the cell is considered damaged, will become arrested in the G_2 stage, and not enter the subsequent phase.

The next and final segment of the cell cycle is known as the M phase. This is where mitosis, or separation of the cell's nucleus into two identical sets containing identical chromosome copies, occurs. The M phase is perhaps the most complex part of the cell cycle and actually involves several distinct stages that are known as prophase, prometaphase, metaphase, anaphase, and telophase (see figure 2).

Prophase involves the consolidation of the nuclear DNA and associated proteins (known as chromatin) into the coiled pieces of DNA (known as chromosomes). Prophase proceeds after DNA replication has occurred. Therefore, there are now two exact copies of each chromosome in the cell, which are termed chromatids. Also within prophase, a component of the cell nucleus called the nucleolus, which is used to transcribe and assemble RNA, dissociates and disappears. Finally, structural components known as centrosomes begin to migrate to opposite poles of the cell and begin to set up a network of cylindrical fibers known as microtubules that will be used to mechanically pull the cell apart.

Following this, cells move into a component of mitosis that is known as prometaphase. During this stage, the membrane surrounding the nucleus begins to deconstruct, leaving visible fragments within the interior of the cell.

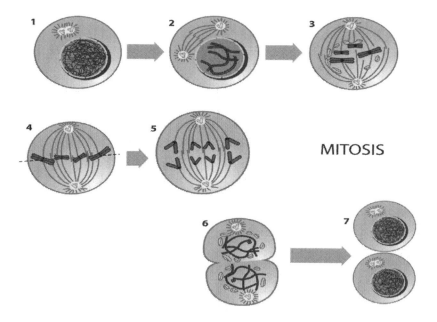

MITOSIS

Figure 2: Mitosis (1) The completion of the G$_2$ phase of the cell cycle marks the end of interphase, after which the process of mitosis begins. (2) The first stage, prophase, is characterized by consolidation of the DNA and early formation of the microtubule apparatus. (3) This is followed by prometaphase, in which kineto-chores are formed, and the kinetochore microtubule apparatus begins to shift the chromosomes to the center of the cell. (4) Metaphase follows, characterized by the alignment of the chromosomes along the metaphase plate that begin to be pulled apart by the spindle apparatus. (5) Anaphase is subsequently marked by complete separation of the chromosomes as they migrate to opposite poles of the cell. (6) In telophase, new nuclei are formed for each daughter cell. (7) In cytokinesis, cellular cytoplasm is formed and divided, resulting in the formation of two identical repli-cas of the original cell.

The chromosomes then form protein constituents known as kineto-chores, which will attach to kinetochore microtubules that stretch from one centrosome to the other on opposite poles of the cell. Prometaphase ends as the microtubules begin to shift the chromosomes to the center of the cell.

As the chromosomes align in the center of the cell and prepare to become separated into the two daughter cells, the stage of mitosis known as metaphase is entered. The alignment occurs at what is known as the metaphase plate, which is an imaginary line that is equidistant from the two centrosomes and involves the attachment of the microtubule fibers to the kinetochores just described. Imagine this as an array of cables attached to two powerful winches on either end of the cell, pulling in opposite directions on an object in the center, with the ultimate goal of drawing it into two equal halves. As metaphase progresses, another cellular checkpoint occurs where appropriate attachment of the kinetochore to the microtubule array must occur before a cell will be allowed to progress on to the next stage.

Following metaphase, the cell moves into anaphase, where the chromosomes actually migrate to opposite ends of the cells. Simultaneously, the microtubule fibers begin to expand the cell, distorting its normal circular shape into that of an oval. This expansion is essential to produce the two daughter cells that are soon to come.

In the final phase of mitosis, known as telophase, the remnant nuclear material of the parent cell envelops each of the daughter cells, thereby creating a new nucleus for each of the daughters. Once situated within this nucleus, the chromosomes unwind to their former chromatin structure. Concomitant with the nucleus formation, a process known as cytokinesis (which is technically distinct from mitosis) takes place, which involves the division of the cellular cytoplasm (the amorphous gel substance outside of the cell nucleus that houses all of the other cellular machinery such as mitochondria) between the two new daughter cells. Once cytokinesis is complete, two identical daughter cells are formed, containing the exact same genetic material as the single parent from which they were derived.

Understanding the laborious process of the cell cycle, we can better appreciate the mechanisms behind the valuable effects of quercetin. Recall that mutations of the p53 gene and proteins are among the most common genetic deformations in human cancer. Quercetin appears to downregulate the expression of p53 proteins to imperceptible concentrations in human breast cancer cell lines in a dose-dependent fashion.[224] This downregulation, in turn, interferes with the cellular replications process, essentially arresting cells at the G_2-M phase of the cell cycle.[225]

Additionally, quercetin's activity through the p53 mechanism appears to affect another stage of the cell cycle. In a study of human leukemia cells, quercetin was found to produce a significant arrest in replication at the G_1 checkpoint described previously.[226] Further, in gastric cancer cells, quercetin administration was found to profoundly reduce cell growth compared to controls not receiving the polyphenol.[227] Much like sentries at the gate, quercetin appears to effectively prevent cancer cells from passing through two pivotal stages of the cell cycle, thereby reducing their ability to proliferate.

In addition to inhibiting key steps within the cell cycle, quercetin has been shown to demonstrate anticarcinogenic activity via other mechanisms. In a study examining prostate cancer cells, researchers discovered that quercetin possesses the ability to promote cellular apoptosis. In this investigation, the flavonoid was determined to downregulate levels of a molecule known as heat shock protein, which has been shown to be an important regulator of cancer cell growth and survival. By decreasing levels of this important cancer promoter, quercetin was found to induce prostate cancer cell apoptosis.[228] As we have seen previously, agents that can promote apoptosis are an important part of the arsenal in cancer treatment, and quercetin's activity here gives promise for its utility as an adjunctive therapy in the oncology space.

In a different type of study, another group of researchers examined the effects of quercetin not only on pro-apoptotic mechanisms, but on anti-proliferation and cancer-cell drug sensitivity as well. Utilizing a pancreatic cancer cell line, investigators in Poland specifically examined the activity of quercetin alone and in combination with a chemotherapy agent known as daunorubicin on the three cancer mechanisms described. With regard to apoptosis, pronounced activity, as expected, was noted with daunorubicin administration. A more modest, but nonetheless significant, effect of quercetin on promoting apoptosis was also identified. Examining pancreatic cancer cell lines known to be sensitive to daunorubicin, quercetin was found to independently inhibit their proliferation and, when administered in combination with daunorubicin, was found to act synergistically with the chemotherapy agent. This is compelling because these findings may allow practitioners to administer a lower dose of the toxic chemotherapy agent if used in combination with quercetin. Finally, quercetin demonstrated an additional benefit by sensitizing a resistant pancreatic cancer cell line to the effects of daunorubicin. In other words, cells that showed no response to daunorubicin alone were destroyed when daunorubicin was administered with quercetin.[229] This trio of effects—pro-apoptotic, anti-proliferative, and cell sensitizing, provide persuasive evidence that quercetin may have significant potential as an adjunctive therapy in cancer treatment.

Moving beyond the laboratory and examining cancer risk and prevention in population studies, it appears that flavonoid ingestion may actually contribute to a reduced risk of developing many types of cancers. We have previously identified a wealth of data on the prevention of colon cancer with a multitude of different natural and pharmacological agents. In this regard, quercetin appears to be no exception. In a case-control study examining 264 patients with confirmed colorectal cancer compared to 408 noncancer controls, researchers in the United Kingdom identified a 50% risk reduction in developing colon cancer with increasing quercetin intake.[230] A similar trend was noted in the Finnish Mobile Clinic Health Examination Survey, which examined a cohort of 62,440 persons. In this study, quercetin intake was stratified by quartile, and those consuming the flavonoid at the highest level demonstrated a 38% risk reduction for the development of colorectal cancer compared to those in the lowest quartile.[231]

In addition to identifying a trend for reduced colorectal cancer incidence with increasing quercetin intake, researchers in the Finnish Mobile Clinic Health Examination Survey revealed a statistically significant overall reduction in any cancer risk of 23% in those in the highest quartile of quercetin intake compared to those in the lowest. When assessed by tissue type, this was driven by a potent reduction in the incidence of lung cancers, which was decreased by an impressive 68% in the group consuming the highest levels of quercetin.[231] A similar trend for reduced lung cancer incidence was identified by researchers in Uruguay in a case-control study involving 541 patients with documented lung cancer who were compared to 540 controls. Results in this series revealed a robust, statistically significant 42% reduction in risk of lung cancer with quercetin intake.[232]

Additional investigations have yielded promising results in other tissue types. In a US study examining pancreatic cancer, quercetin intake, as part of a diet rich in other flavonols as well, was associated with a reduced risk for pancreatic cancer in a cohort of smokers.[233] Similarly, in a study known as the Alpha-Tocopherol, Beta-Carotene Cancer Prevention Study, those subjects who were randomized to placebo (i.e., not taking the experimental supplements of alpha-tocopherol and/or beta-carotene), but analyzed by quercetin intake demonstrated a 64% reduction in pancreatic cancer risk in the highest quartile of flavonol consumption compared to the lowest.[234] Data from the same study also revealed a similar risk reduction in the same male smoker cohort for the development of renal cell carcinoma, with those in the top quartile of quercetin ingestion demonstrating a 40% reduction in risk for developing the malignancy compared to their counterparts in the lowest tier.[235] We have much more to learn about the activity of quercetin and other flavonoids in the oncology arena, but multiple lines of evidence support an anticancer role for these natural compounds. Case-control evidence provides compelling insight into cancer risk reduction with these potent antimicroinflammatory agents, and combining this with the robust laboratory data in the anti-proliferative, pro-apoptotic, and tumor-sensitizing arenas, there is provocative rationale for incorporating quercetin as an adjunctive agent in the treatment of cancer.

Looking at quercetin's specific activity in the microinflammatory arena, there is abundant evidence supporting its activity in key pathways. In cellular analyses, quercetin demonstrates the ability to block IL-8 activation as well as its gene expression induced by TNF-α.[236] In another experiment assessing the release of cytokines from human mast cells, quercetin inhibited the release of IL-6, IL-8, and TNF-α by 82%–93%![237] In macrophages, low concentrations of quercetin have been shown to induce the production of IL-10, an important antimicroinflammatory and regulatory cytokine.[238] In a population of stimulated nerve cells known as astrocytes, quercetin has been shown to decrease elevated levels of familiar proinflammatory substances, including IL-6, IL-8, and MCP-1.[239] Finally, in what has been previously demonstrated as a critical component of the microinflammatory pathways, quercetin has demonstrated potent inhibition of NF-ϰB activity.[240] Without question, this powerful flavonoid demonstrates significant activity on multiple microinflammatory fronts, paving a clear path to its utility in the forefront of battling inflammation-based pathways.

This brings us to the activity of quercetin in cardiovascular disease, which, by now, we have readily identified as a prototypical microinflammatory disease. We have seen that one of the early pathophysiological processes critical to the evolution of atherosclerosis is the oxidation of the LDL cholesterol molecule so that it becomes more "appetizing" to the macrophages and can be used to build the atherosclerotic plaque. Quercetin has been shown to inhibit the peroxidation process that is crucial for converting LDL into its atherogenic form, thereby demonstrating the potential to retard plaque formation essentially at its origin.[241]

In addition to inhibiting peroxidation of the LDL molecule, quercetin functions in other antioxidant capacities that are important in coronary physiology. Quercetin, similar to many flavonoids, is a potent scavenger of many reactive oxygen species, including superoxide, hydroxyl, and peroxyl radicals.[242,243] This antioxidant function is significant, because by reducing reactive oxygen species concentrations—particularly superoxide—quercetin increases nitric oxide availability and enhances its activity.[244] Recall, nitric oxide is a key player in cardiovascular physiology, critical in maintaining normal endothelial function. By protecting nitric oxide function from harmful reactive oxygen species, quercetin and other flavonoids create a potent defense against oxidative insults and promote a healthier endothelium that can resist atherosclerotic transformation.

As we have previously seen, elevated blood pressure is a potent risk factor for the development of atherosclerotic disease, and several investigations have examined the effect of quercetin in patients with high blood pressure. These studies were predicated on the foundation that diets rich in fruits and vegetables—major sources of flavonoids—were associated with decreased blood pressure.[245] Moreover, laboratory investigations demonstrate that quercetin has important vasodilatory effects in isolated arteries (an important effect in normalizing blood pressure) and actually reduces blood pressure in hypertensive rats.[246,247] Most compelling, however, a randomized, double-blind, placebo-controlled study conducted by investigators from the University of Utah in prehypertensive and hypertensive men and women reveals that quercetin supplementation produces a statistically significant reduction in blood pressure in patients with preexisting hypertension.[248] This powerful effect of quercetin is a landmark finding and supports its efficacy in modulating coronary risk by treating one of the prominent accelerators of the atherosclerotic process—hypertension.

Clinically, in addition to attenuating cardiac risk by reducing blood pressure, quercetin and other flavonoids have demonstrated efficacy in reducing other processes that contribute to pathophysiological manifestations of coronary artery disease. We have previously identified the deleterious effects of matrix metalloproteinase enzymes in degrading and making unstable the fibrous cap that houses the atherosclerotic plaque. Quercetin and its flavonoid cousins appear to reduce the expression of at least two matrix metalloproteinases, MMP-2 and MMP-9.[249] Additionally, flavonoids appear to inhibit platelet aggregation, an important process that leads to heart attack when an unstable coronary plaque ruptures.[250,251] Finally, patients with coronary artery disease taking flavonol-rich juice or tea demonstrate increases in coronary vasodilation, an important protective mechanism to maximize blood flow to the heart muscle that is frequently disrupted when the endothelium is dysfunctional.[252,253] Given these critical clinical effects, quercetin has the potential to play an important role in reducing risk for the development of, and decreasing adverse consequences of, atherosclerotic coronary artery disease.

A plethora of data exists purporting the beneficial effects of plant-derived polyphenols in risk reduction and treatment of cancer and coronary disease. The mechanisms detailed previously demonstrate exciting revelations in understanding the antimicroinflammatory activities of these agents at the cellular and molecular level and give promise to their utility in disease prevention and management. Without question, more study is needed to realize the full potential of these substances, but enough evidence already exists supporting the utility of these potent, natural plant-derived agents. We look forward to exciting new research in this arena that will hopefully expand the clinical function of these promising substances in the fight against cancer, coronary, and other diseases.

OTHER AGENTS WITH ANTIMICROINFLAMMATORY ACTIVITY
Omega-3 Fatty Acids

Omega-3 fatty acids, also known as omega-3 long chain polyunsaturated fatty acids (PUFAs), n-3 polyunsaturated fatty acids, or simply omega-3 fish oils, are a group of fats that are commonly found in plant oils, marine plants, and marine animals. They are considered essential fatty acids, which, like essential vitamins or minerals, are needed for fundamental functions within our bodies, but are not produced by our normal metabolic processes. As a result, we must ingest these fatty acids from exogenously derived sources on a regular basis in order to meet certain of our physiological requirements. The most common sources of omega-3 fatty acids are fish oils, which are abundant in fatty fish such as trout, chub, salmon, albacore tuna, mackerel, sardines, and herring. Certain plant oils, such as flaxseed oil, have very high concentrations of omega-3 fatty acids, with lesser, but still significant, amounts being present in canola and soybean oils. Algae also constitute another source of omega-3 fatty acids and are commonly ingested for their nutritional value in vegan diets. Certain nuts also contain significant amounts of omega-3 fatty acids, with the highest concentrations being present in walnuts.

It is useful to examine a quantitative framework for the nutritional value of these different omega-3-containing food sources to understand how they compare to one another. The fish with the highest concentrations of total omega-3 fatty acids are led by lake trout, followed by chub, Atlantic mackerel, and herring, which contain 4.6, 2.6, 2.6, and 2.5 grams of omega-3 fatty acids per 100 grams of edible tissue, respectively. Many people regard salmon as possessing the highest concentrations of omega-3 fats, but looking at Atlantic, chinook, coho, and sockeye varieties, they only contain 1.8, 1.4, 1.2, and 1.2 grams of omega-3 per 100 grams of edible meat.[254,255] Examining flaxseed oil, approximately 1 tablespoon of the plant derivative provides about 6 to 7 grams of omega-3 PUFAs. Soybeans, as another plant source, provide approximately 3.2 grams of omega-3 fats per 100 grams of soybeans, placing them in a higher concentration than many fish species. Astoundingly, the list of omega-3 sources is led by walnuts, which provide a hefty 10.4 grams of the fatty acid per 100 grams of edible nuts![256]

Not all omega-3 fatty acids are created equal, however, and it is important to understand the differences in the specific type of omega-3 PUFAs that can be ingested. There are three principal omega-3 fatty acids, which are known as alpha-linolenic acid (ALA), eicosapentaenoic acid (EPA), and docosahexaenoic acid (DHA). The most common sources of ALA in the human diet are plant oils, whereas the principal sources of EPA and DHA are fish. Algae oil almost exclusively provides DHA. The least usable form of omega-3 fatty acid within the human body is ALA, which, once ingested, can actually be converted to small amounts of both EPA and DHA. As a result, one must use caution when examining omega-3 sources and understand, for example, that despite its overall high concentration of omega-3 fats, flaxseed oil is principally ALA, which must be converted following ingestion to more usable EPA and DHA forms to meet our nutritional demands.[257,258]

Before discussing the benefits of omega-3 fatty acids, it is important to spotlight a related group of fats known as the omega-6 fatty acids. The news and literature are filled with information regarding the importance of balancing the ingestion of omega-3 and omega-6 PUFAs. Omega-6 fats are found largely in meats and processed foods, and most experts would agree that the typical Western diet is heavy in omega-6 fatty acid intake. In fact, reports indicate that the American diet contains at least fifteen times more omega-6 fatty acid intake than omega-3.[259] There is controversy among nutritional authorities, however, regarding the exact tenets of balancing these two fatty acids. Some experts assert that the excess in omega-6 fatty acids typical of a Western diet contributes to many chronic disease states, whereas others do not believe the ratio is significant at all. Keeping this in mind, we will explore the science behind the health benefits of omega-3 fatty acids, and only highlight relevant data regarding the adverse effects of omega-6 PUFAs without attempting to resolve the debate on the appropriate balance between these two dietary fats.

The efficacy of omega-3 fatty acids in the prevention and/or management of a host of diseases, including cancer and atherosclerosis, has been analyzed extensively over the previous couple of decades. Moreover, omega-3 fats have been used to treat many other conditions, from psychiatric illness to developmental disorders and macroinflammatory diseases such as arthritis. We will focus our attention on the utility of omega-3 fatty acids in the microinflammatory arena and their ability to attenuate processes that promote cancer, coronary disease, and aging.

As we have illustrated with many of the nutritional supplements described in this chapter, one of the initial steps in analyzing the efficacy of a nutraceutical in the microinflammatory arena is demonstrating that it can positively affect the levels of established microinflammatory markers. Omega-3 PUFAs have been examined extensively in this regard, with an abundance of data demonstrating that they can indeed affect levels of familiar biomarkers of microinflammation. Beginning with CRP, several lines of evidence suggest that regular ingestion of omega-3 fatty acids can reduce levels of this microinflammatory surrogate. In a small, randomized crossover study (type of study where subjects are initiallygiven one type of treatment, followed by a washout period where no therapy is administered, then concluded with a second type of treatment . This type of investigation allows researchers to assess the effect of two or more therapies in the same individual) assessing omega-3 PUFA supplementation in diabetics, researchers discovered significant effects of omega-3 ingestion on CRP concentrations. As one would expect, serum levels of EPA and DHA were elevated at the four-week and twelve-week marks in subjects receiving the omega-3 supplements. More importantly, CRP levels were significantly decreased in the active treatment groups, confirming the efficacy of the omega-3 fatty acids in reducing this important marker of microinflammation.[260]

In another series that assessed the efficacy of omega-3 supplementation on reducing CRP levels in a population of exercise-trained men, researchers found similar results. In this investigation, similar to the previous, subjects were randomized in a double-blind crossover fashion to six weeks of therapy with omega-3 PUFAs, followed by an eight-week washout period. As expected, during treatment with the fatty acid supplements, subjects demonstrated statistically significant elevations in blood levels of EPA and DHA. Moreover, under active omega-3 treatment, test subjects demonstrated statistically significant reductions in CRP levels compared to their placebo counterparts.[261] In a different population with a similarly designed crossover study, omega-3 PUFAs again appear efficacious in reducing microinflammatory markers.

In another research study, investigators examined the effect of omega-3 supplementation on markers of microinflammation in healthy older adults. In this examination, subjects were given an eight-week experimental diet consisting of a combination of fatty fish and sardine oil, with measurement of serum markers of microinflammation appropriately performed before and after active treatment. A statistically significant reduction in serum C-reactive protein levels compared to baseline values was identified following the eight-week treatment period.[262] This and the previous study confirm that relatively short periods of treatment with omega-3 PUFAs can produce significant impacts on CRP as a marker of the microinflammatory process.

In each of the previous investigations, patients were not required to have baseline elevations in CRP. Rather, researchers simply compared reference levels of the microinflammatory marker to that obtained following the specified omega-3 treatment protocol. In another series, researchers specifically analyzed the effect of omega-3 PUFAs on patients with baseline elevations of CRP. In this study, which was a randomized, placebo-controlled investigation that did not include a crossover protocol, subjects with high reference concentrations of CRP received eight weeks of treatment with either omega-3 supplements or placebo. Compared to placebo, those subjects receiving omega-3 PUFAs demonstrated a robust 40% reduction in CRP levels that was highly statistically significant.[263] This is compelling data in the face of a study population already at risk for adverse consequences based upon elevations of the microinflammatory marker CRP! Many additional investigations identify similar findings, yielding provocative evidence that omega-3 long chain polyunsaturated fatty acids can attenuate levels of microinflammatory markers.

Examining other biomarkers of microinflammation, there is also a plethora of data regarding the effect of omega-3 PUFAs on the key inflammatory cytokine TNF-α. In one series that examined type 2 diabetic patients, researchers conducted a double-blind, placebo-controlled trial assessing the effect of omega-3 fatty acids on serum levels of inflammatory markers in this high-risk population. Participants were administered daily doses of either placebo, which was sunflower oil, or the study supplement, a mixture of EPA and DHA, for eight weeks. Microinflammatory biomarker measurements were taken at baseline and at study termination. As expected, the placebo group demonstrated no significant change in markers of microinflammation following eight weeks of sunflower oil administration. However, those subjects receiving the omega-3 fatty acids demonstrated statistically significant reductions in TNF-α levels.[264]

In another study assessing the antimicroinflammatory effect of omega-3 supplementation in a chronic congestive heart failure population, researchers compared the action of omega-3 PUFAs to placebo on markers of heart failure and microinflammation. Patients were randomized to the omega-3 supplement or placebo for a treatment duration of three months, and values of microinflammatory markers were compared between the two groups at baseline and at the end of the protocol interval. The omega-3-PUFA-treated group demonstrated a potent reduction in TNF-α compared to placebo that was highly significant.[265]

In a separate protocol examining the effect of omega-3 fatty acids on microinflammatory markers in healthy volunteer subjects, researchers compared the effects of four weeks of flaxseed oil administration to a four-week regimen of flaxseed and fish oil combined. The primary end point was the cellular production of TNF-α in the two treatment phases compared to baseline levels. Subjects taking the initial four weeks of flaxseed oil demonstrated a prominent and statistically significant 30% reduction in TNF-α production. Furthermore, after the fish oil was added for an additional four weeks, TNF-α levels were reduced by an impressive 74%.[266] This data demonstrates two compelling pieces of evidence: (1) both flaxseed oil and fish oil can produce significant reductions in microinflammatory biomarkers, and (2) the magnitude of biomarker reduction is much more pronounced with fish oil compared to flaxseed oil. As we iterated previously, not all omega-3 PUFAs are equivalent, and this investigation appears to confirm that adage and suggests that fish-derived PUFAs are more effective at reducing microinflammatory markers. In any case, based upon this and the other studies we have discussed, it does appear that omega-3 fatty acids are effectual at reducing the microinflammatory marker TNF-α in multiple populations.

Since TNF-α and CRP represent only two of many biomarkers of inflammation, is there data supporting omega-3 fatty acid efficacy in reducing other microinflammatory surrogates? Indeed, multiple lines of investigation have assessed other typical microinflammation markers and seem to demonstrate that PUFAs can reduce these as well. In the same trial just outlined, investigators not only examined the effect of the omega-3 supplements on TNF-α. They also analyzed the ability of PUFAs to decrease interleukin-1 beta (IL-1 beta) as well. After the initial four weeks of the protocol, which incorporated a flaxseed oil–based regimen, IL-1 beta production was decreased to a similar extent as TNF-α—approximately 30%. In the second phase, where fish oil supplements were added for an additional four weeks, IL-1 beta levels were, again, similar to TNF-α levels, reduced significantly more at 80%.[266] This is a compelling demonstration of the extent to which omega-3 fatty acids can reduce microinflammatory biomarkers, and highlights what may be a fundamental difference in efficacy between plant-derived and fish-derived PUFAs.

Another noteworthy example of the effect of omega-3 fatty acids on microinflammatory indices involves the cellular adhesion molecules, which we have seen in the atherosclerotic process. Older studies established that omega-3 PUFAs could interfere with the metabolism of both vascular cell adhesion molecule 1 (VCAM-1) and intercellular adhesion molecule 1 (ICAM-I).[267,268] Moreover, a recently published meta-analysis assessed eighteen different clinical trials that addressed the relationship between

PUFA supplementation and the plasma concentrations of the microinflammatory biomarker soluble intercellular adhesion molecule 1 (sICAM-1). Investigators identified a statistically significant reduction in sICAM-1 in the aggregate of test subjects, but, more interestingly, found the same reduction when stratifying patients with and without abnormal serum cholesterol profiles.[269] This powerful data again demonstrates that in heterogeneous test populations, supplementation with omega-3 fatty acids can significantly reduce microinflammatory indicators, and this effect does not require the presence of microinflammation-inciting disease processes such as abnormal cholesterol.

From a clinical perspective, omega-3 fatty acid supplements have demonstrated a wide range of utility in the disease management arena. Many people are likely aware of the use of fish oils in the management of cardiovascular disease, as this has been highlighted in the media for many years. However, most individuals are probably not aware of the utilization of omega-3 PUFAs in cancer treatment, as this has not been as well publicized. We will explore the use of these natural agents in both of these microinflammatory-based disease processes.

Omega-3 fatty acids have slowly developed greater popularity in the realm of cardiovascular disease management as the last decade has witnessed a wealth of rigorous investigation by cardiovascular disease authorities worldwide. The most recent update to the American Heart Association/American College of Cardiology Foundation guidelines for the secondary prevention and risk reduction of patients with atherosclerotic disease was published in 2011 and provided a recommendation that for "all patients, it may be reasonable to recommend omega-3 fatty acids from fish or fish oil capsules (1g/d) for cardiovascular disease risk reduction."[270] This endorsement by the leading cardiovascular societies in the United States testifies to the plethora of data that has highlighted the efficacy of fish oil treatment in this arena. We will examine the data that has provided the foundation for this compelling endorsement.

Fish oil's ability to reduce cardiovascular disease risk was, like many treatments we have examined thus far, rooted in epidemiological data. In a series of studies published in the 1980s and 1990s, fish consumption in heterogeneous populations was associated with a significantly lower mortality in the study subjects than those who consumed no fish at all.[271-273] A more recent evaluation conducted as part of the Nurses' Health Study demonstrated similar findings in women, with a decremental risk of developing coronary heart disease noted with increasing levels of fish consumption or omega-3 supplement intake.[274] Most compelling, however, a large meta-analysis of multiple cohort studies was published in 2004 and incorporated data from eleven studies with a combined population of 222,364 patients with an average of almost twelve years of follow-up. Similar to the data in the Nurses' Health Study, this meta-analysis demonstrated a progressive decrease in coronary heart disease mortality with increasing levels of fish consumption. Quantitatively, investigators determined that coronary mortality was reduced by 11% for fish consumption of one to three times per month, 85% for consumption once per week, 23% for consumption two to four times per week, and a potent 38% for consumption of fish five or more times per week. Aggregated, this translated to a 7% reduction in coronary heart disease mortality for each 20 gram/day increase in fish intake.[275] In diverse and large patient populations, these epidemiological evaluations provide convincing evidence that fish oil and/or fish consumption can reduce the risk of developing coronary artery disease and reduce cardiac mortality.

Moving from observational series and meta-analyses, a wealth of data from randomized, controlled trials is available and further supports the utility of omega-3 fatty acids in the management of cardiovascular disease.

The first randomized trial assessing omega-3 PUFAs in patients with established coronary artery disease was known as the Diet and Reinfarction Trial (DART). In this investigation, 2,033 men who survived initial heart attacks were randomized, following recovery, to one of three dietary modifications that consisted of: (1) reducing fat intake and increasing the ratio of polyunsaturated to saturated fat, (2) increasing fatty fish consumption, and (3) increasing cereal fiber intake. The individuals in the group who increased their intake of fatty fish demonstrated a statistically significant 29% reduction in all-cause mortality after two years, compared to the individuals who did not receive advice on increased fish consumption.[276] This mortality benefit is certainly impressive, but another provocative point illustrated by this trial was that it did not take much of an increase in fatty fish consumption to confer such a protective effect. Quantitatively, the benefit was seen with only an increase of about 300 grams of fish per week, corresponding to approximately 2.5 grams of EPA![276] As a result, these data are not only impressive regarding the mortality reduction, but also suggest that even modest increases in our PUFA intake can produce important health benefits.

Another trial took DART one step further and prospectively randomized patients to either fish oil capsules, mustard oil capsules, or placebo immediately on hospital admission for suspected heart attacks. In this trial, patients received considerably more fish oil equivalents than those in the DART trial, as each capsule, which was taken daily, provided a total of 1.6 grams of EPA and DHA. After one year of follow-up, total cardiac event rates were 25% in the fish oil group, a value that was significantly lower than the 35% event rate in the placebo cohort.[277] As a result, this provided mounting evidence that omega-3 fatty acid administration has a powerful role in the secondary prevention of those initially presenting with cardiac events.

A final trial worth discussing that truly hits home the benefit of omega-3 fatty acid in preventing recurrent cardiovascular events in coronary disease patients is known as the GISSI (Gruppo Italiano per lo Studio della Sopravvivenza nell'Infarto Miocardico) Prevention Study. In this investigation, over eleven thousand patients with known coronary heart disease already receiving standard therapy were randomized to 850 milligrams of EPA and DHA, 300 milligrams of vitamin E, both, or neither. Patients were followed for three and a half years, after which analysis of the data revealed that those receiving the fish oil alone had a robust and statistically significant 15% reduction in the combined primary end point of death, nonfatal myocardial infarction (heart attack) and nonfatal stroke. Moreover, this group demonstrated an equally significant 20% reduction in all-cause mortality, as well as a powerful 45% reduction in sudden cardiac death![278] Based upon these series, it appears that omega-3 fatty acids produce significant benefit with regard to standard cardiovascular end points in patients with known coronary artery disease.

Examining atherosclerotic disease in another way, investigators from the University of Munich in Germany conducted a randomized, double-blind, placebo-controlled trial assessing the effect of omega-3 fatty acids on progression of coronary atherosclerosis. Coronary atherosclerosis was assessed by angiography (a procedure where catheters are placed in the coronary arteries and contrast is injected in order to illuminate the arteries and measure the cholesterol plaque) at enrollment and two years later. Patients were randomized to receive either placebo or fish oil concentrate, which was administered at a dose of 6 grams per day for three months, then 3 grams per day for twenty-one months. Results of the study revealed that subjects taking fish oil supplements demonstrated significantly less progression, as well as more regression, in atherosclerotic plaque burden compared to placebo.[279] This type of information is quite compelling because it provides an anatomic correlate to the clinical end points identified in the prior trials, adding a more global perspective to understanding the efficacy of omega-3 fatty acids in treating atherosclerotic coronary artery disease.

A different type of anatomic study assessed the effect of omega-3 fish oil supplements on preventing early closure of bypass grafts in patients who had undergone coronary bypass surgery. In this investigation, researchers randomized 610 patients undergoing coronary artery bypass graft surgery to receive standard treatment (at that time, this was blood thinning with aspirin or warfarin) or standard therapy plus 4 grams per day of fish oil. At one year, patients received angiography of the bypass grafts to assess whether or not they remained open In those patients receiving fish oil supplements, bypass grafts were found to be closed less frequently at a rate of 27% compared to 33% for those receiving standard therapy alone.[280] This difference reached statistical significance, and, once again provided another line of confirmatory evidence in favor of the antiatherosclerotic properties of omega-3 fatty acids.

Although there are some trials demonstrating no significant benefit of omega-3 PUFAs on cardiovascular end points, the aggregate data appear to support the efficacy of these agents in reducing cardiac events and preventing disease progression. This net positive benefit is the principal reason that omega-3 fatty acids are included as therapeutic options in the most recent iteration of the American Heart Association/American College of Cardiology guidelines. Given the strong microinflammatory basis of atherosclerotic coronary artery disease, and the anti-inflammatory properties of the omega-3 fatty acids, it is no surprise that these natural substances should be added to our armamentarium in the fight against coronary atherosclerosis.

Beyond their direct effects on atherosclerosis, it is noteworthy that studies have revealed other properties of omega-3 PUFAs that directly impact cardiovascular disease development and progression. As we have discussed, high blood pressure is an important risk factor in atherosclerotic coronary artery disease, and treating it to normal levels is critical to maintaining cardiovascular health and preventing heart attacks and strokes. Several studies have demonstrated that omega-3 fatty acids can produce a small, but measurable decrease in blood pressure. In one meta-analysis of seventeen controlled clinical trials with average omega-3 fatty acid supplementation of greater than 3 grams a day, investigators determined that in patients with both treated and previously untreated high blood pressure, omega-3 supplementation could produce clinically relevant blood pressure reductions.[281] Similarly, in a separate meta-analysis of thirty-one placebo-controlled trials that examined a dose-response effect of omega-3 supplementation on blood pressure control, investigators delineated a statistically significant dose-related increase in blood pressure reduction with higher levels of omega-3 fatty acid intake.[282] Together, these important studies demonstrate that in a large pool of hypertensive patients, omega-3 PUFAs appear to produce relevant blood pressure reductions, highlighting a potential ancillary benefit of these agents in the prevention of adverse cardiovascular outcomes.

In addition to reducing blood pressure, PUFAs appear to decrease cardiovascular risk by inhibiting certain coagulation parameters. Omega-3 fatty acids have been shown to reduce platelet aggregation—one of the critical processes that leads to clot formation within the coronary arteries during a heart attack.[283,284] Additionally, other investigation has revealed that omega-3 fatty acids may actually augment a process known as fibrinolysis, which is a protective action that breaks up clots within our blood vessels.[285,286] The combined effect of omega-3 fish oils to both inhibit one of the initial steps in clot formation and promote the dissolution of clots after they have been created is a potentially valuable adjunct in the fight against coronary artery disease and its adverse consequences.

Perhaps the most impressive effect of omega-3 fatty acids outside of direct microinflammatory inhibition is their ability to dramatically reduce serum triglycerides. As previously discussed, one of the defining features of the metabolic syndrome is elevation in circulating fats, or triglycerides, which are an independent risk factor for coronary heart disease. Studies have revealed that relatively large doses of omega-3 fatty acids derived from fish oil (4 grams a day) can produce profound reductions in serum triglyceride levels of approximately 26%–47%, with concomitant elevations in good cholesterol (HDL) of about 11%–14%.[287,288] Given these profound effects, a prescription formulation of omega-3 fatty acids was produced and is currently available for physicians to prescribe to their patients with primary triglyceride elevations. An important consideration here, however, is that despite the positive effect of high doses of omega-3 fatty acids on triglycerides and HDL cholesterol, clinical trials have demonstrated that they can produce a 10%–46% increase in bad cholesterol (LDL) as well.[288] As a result, it is important for individuals to consult with their physicians on the appropriate dosage of omega-3 fatty acids, since, as we have pointed out on previous topics, more is not necessarily always better.

Research in the last two to three decades has clearly established a role for omega-3 fatty acids in the prevention and management of atherosclerotic coronary artery disease. As we have seen, a wealth of data supports the antimicroinflammatory efficacy of these agents, which seems to be one of the foundational properties of these supplements in cardiovascular risk reduction. Furthermore, the ancillary effects of omega-3 PUFAs in reducing blood pressure, preventing platelet aggregation, inducing fibrinolysis, and decreasing serum triglyceride levels enhances their potency for global cardiovascular protection. Ongoing research continues to explore this powerful nature-derived therapy and will hopefully elucidate many more clinical applications for omega-3 fatty acids within the cardiovascular disease treatment arena.

Beyond coronary artery disease, omega-3 fatty acids appear to have efficacy in modulating cancer risk in certain tissue types. We previously mentioned that we would avoid the controversy between omega-3 PUFAs and omega-6 PUFAs, but, as these agents relate to cancer and carcinogenesis, some important data has been identified regarding both types of dietary fats and we will explore relevant information in this regard.

Several recently published epidemiological studies assessing diverse demographicshave demonstrated a positive association between omega-6 fatty acid intake and breast cancer risk. In one series known as the Singapore Chinese Health Study, 35,298 women were analyzed as part of a 63,257 person cohort. Patients were followed and stratified into quartiles of dietary intake based upon consumption of omega-3 and omega-6 PUFAs. Those women consuming the highest levels of omega-3 fatty acids demonstrated a significantly lower, a 26% reduction in, risk of breast cancer compared to those in the lowest quartile of intake. Moreover, women who simultaneously consumed low levels of omega-3 PUFAs and high levels of omega-6 PUFAs demonstrated a strongly significant increased risk of developing advanced-stage breast cancer compared to those who consumed both low levels of omega-6 and omega-3 PUFAs.[289] This provocative analysis not only supports the beneficial effects of omega-3 fatty acids in reducing breast cancer risk, but suggest that an abundance of omega-6 fatty acids can increase risk for developing a potentially fatal cancer.

In another series examining women in France, investigators analyzed 74,524 subjects between the years of 1993 and 2002, stratifying them in quintiles of omega-6 and omega-3 PUFA intake. Unlike the Singapore Chinese Health Study, results from this French investigation demonstrated no independent increase in risk of breast cancer based upon increased omega-3 fatty acid intake. However, similar to the Singapore study, women with a combined low intake of omega-3 PUFAs and high intake of omega-6 PUFAs did demonstrate a statistically significant increase in risk for developing breast cancer.[290] Again, this is compelling epidemiological evidence of the adverse effects of increased omega-6 fatty acid consumption and supports proponents who believe that the relative balance between omega-6 and omega-3 fatty acids is more important than the absolute consumption of one or the other.

This concept of the interaction between omega-6 and omega-3 PUFAs was further supported by another prospective cohort study known as the Shanghai Women's Health Study. In this investigation, PUFA consumption was analyzed in a group of 72,571 Chinese women. Investigators again found no independent association of breast cancer with omega-3 or omega-6 fatty acid intake. However, they did identify a statistically significant interaction between omega-6 and omega-3 consumption and increased breast cancer risk. Similar to the previous two trials, women who concomitantly ingested the lowest levels of omega-3 PUFAs and highest levels of omeg-6 PUFAs had a markedly increased chance of developing breast cancer compared to those who had the highest intake of omega-3 and lowest intake of omega-6 fatty acids.[291] As a result, this large prospective cohort evaluation corroborates the notion that the relative consumption of omega-6 PUFAs to omega-3 PUFAs may be a more significant consideration than the dietary consumption of either one individually.

Taking these provocative insights one step further, investigators recently reported a population-based case-control study among Mexican women, relating breast cancer risk to both polyunsaturated fatty acid ingestion and obesity. In this series, 1,000 women with breast cancer were examined vis-à-vis 1,074 matched control subjects without breast cancer. Patients were stratified by body mass index as well as intake of omega-6 PUFAs and omega-3 PUFAs.. Unlike the previous series, investigators identified a statistically significant increase in risk for developing breast cancer with increasing levels of omega-6 fatty acid consumption. Moreover, they also identified a statistically decreased risk of breast cancer with increasing omega-3 PUFAs exclusive to obese women, which was not present in those stratified to the normal body weight or overweight groups. This previously undocumented association led investigators to speculate that the underlying protective effect of omega-3 PUFAs in obese women may be related to "decreased inflammation and improved adipokin and estrogen levels induced by omega-3 PUFA in adipose tissue in obese women."[292] Such findings are clearly consistent with our prior discussion of the mechanisms of obesity in microinflammation and the manner in which this contributes to both atherosclerotic and cancer risk.

Although the debate between absolute ingestion of omega-3 and omega-6 PUFAs versus the relative proportions of these two fatty acids is far from resolved, these data undoubtedly demonstrate that there is likely an increased risk for breast cancer in those consuming higher levels of omega-6 PUFAs, and there may be a protective effect in women ingesting increased concentrations of omega-3 fatty acids. The microinflammatory connection elucidated in the Mexican case-control study is an exciting revelation and illuminates the need to further explore the mechanisms underlying PUFA physiology. Indeed, a wealth of research regarding these mechanisms has emerged over the past decade, and we will examine the available evidence supporting the microinflammatory interaction of both omega-3 and omega-6 fatty acids in carcinogenesis.

We have previously discussed the microinflammatory cyclooxygenase and lipoxygenase pathways and their importance in the low-grade inflammatory processes that contribute to aging, cancer, and coronary disease. The principal substrate of both of these pathways is arachidonic acid, which is primarily produced from a fatty acid known as linoleic acid, the most prevalent omega-6 PUFA in the Western diet. It is well established that the 5-lipoxygenase (LOX) enzyme system converts arachidonic acid to a host of microinflammatory mediators that are associated with cardiovascular disease and other conditions characterized by chronic inflammation.[293]

Moreover, several investigations have implicated the LOX system in tumor development and progression in multiple tissue types, including colon, prostate, pancreas, and breast.[294-297]

An interesting investigation into the direct association of omega-6 PUFAs, lipoxygenase and breast cancer risk was published in 2008 and involved a provocative population-based case-control examination of women with a genetic defect in the 5-lipoxygenase (LOX) enzyme system. Investigators discovered that among a group of ethnically diverse women from the San Francisco Bay Area with genetic aberrations in the LOX enzyme system who consumed the highest levels of linoleic acid, there was a profound, 80%, increase in the risk of breast cancer compared to those with the same LOX defect who consumed lower concentrations of omega-6 PUFAs.[298] This genetic-dietary interaction is not only a powerful testament to the significance of the interplay between our genetic predispositions and environmental influences that can provoke disease, but a lucid example of the potentially harmful effects of omega-6 fatty acids.

Another compelling aspect of fatty acids in breast cancer relates to the presence of fatigue in breast cancer survivors, the potential relationship between fatigue and microinflammation, and the ability of omega-3 and omega-6 fatty acids to modify this microinflammatory activity. Among women who survive breast cancer, fatigue is a relatively common symptom and may persist for years after successful treatment.[299] Clinical investigations have suggested that this fatigue is actually propagated by increased cytokine and stress hormone production that ultimately produces a microinflammatory state.[300-302] We have previously established that increased omega-3 PUFA intake is associated with decreased microinflammatory biomarkers, but it is also evident that an elevated ratio of omega-6 to omega-3 PUFAs is coupled to an increase in microinflammatory markers, including IL-1, IL-6, CRP, and TNF-α.[303,304]

Given this foundation, a recently published investigation examined the interplay between fatigue, microinflammation, and the relative ingestion of omega-6 and omega-3 fatty acids in women who survived breast cancer treatment. Investigators identified an escalation in fatigue scores among subjects with increasing levelsof CRP such that those with elevated CRP had a statistically significant 1.8 times greater odds of having fatigue compared to those with lower CRP concentrations. Moreover, subjects who ingested higher levels of omega-6 relative to omega-3 PUFAs demonstrated a profound increase in fatigue compared to those with a lower relative omega-6 intake. Finally, women consuming a lower proportion of omega-3 to omega-6 fatty acids demonstrated a dramatic 4.5 times increased odds of having a high-risk CRP level compared to those ingesting the highest proportion of omega-3 to omega-6 fatty acids.[305] These new insights into the relationship between microinflammation, fatigue, and fatty acid intake bring to light another potentially important target for antimicroinflammatory treatment and highlight the multidimensionality of chronic low-grade inflammatory processes within our bodies.

Beyond the wealth of data that link omega-3 and omega-6 fatty acid consumption to different facets of breast cancer risk, there is a plethora of investigation examining these PUFAs in other types of tumors. In an older trial conducted among men living in a veterans home in Los Angeles, investigators randomized subjects to a diet high in omega-6 PUFAs versus one low in saturated fats and cholesterol for approximately eight and a half years. The group ingesting higher levels of polyunsaturated fat had a significantly higher rate of fatal and nonfatal cancers involving multiple organ systems, including the oropharynx, stomach, lung, and prostate.[306] Other trials investigating the risk of omega-6 intake and cancers in different anatomic sites have been less conclusive, but the preponderance of evidence does not seem to support an increased risk of other types of cancer with increasing omega-6 PUFA ingestion.

On the other hand, many trials demonstrate a potential chemoprotective or chemopreventive role for omega-3 fatty acids. In a large prospective, population-based study conducted in Japan, investigators analyzed subjects through an average nine-year assessment period with regard to incidence of colorectal carcinoma and intake of omega-3 and omega-6 fatty acids. This study was the first to stratify patients by cancer location within either the colon or rectum (most studies lump these anatomic locations together as colorectal cancer), and researchers failed to disclose a relationship between absolute or relative omega-3 and omega-6 ingestion and rectal cancer. However, they did identify a statistically significant decrease in risk for developing colon cancer in subjects within the highest quintile of omega-3 PUFA intake compared to the lowest quintile.[307]

Similar results were observed in a recently published meta-analysis of fourteen prospective cohort trials that demonstrated patients consuming the highest levels of fatty fish had a 12% reduction in relative risk of colorectal cancer compared to those in the groups with the lowest levels of fatty fish ingestion.[308] A separate case-control study examining 929 patients with colorectal cancer compared to 943 matched cancer-free controls demonstrated a robust 39% risk reduction for those in the highest quartile of omega-3 PUFA intake compared to the lowest.[309] Finally, in another study that examined serum PUFA levels in patients undergoing colonoscopy, researchers discovered a 33% reduction in colorectal adenomas in the group with the highest serum omega-3 PUFA levels compared to the lowest. Interestingly, investigators also disclosed a 68% increased risk for developing adenomas in subjects with the highest serum levels of omega-6 PUFAs compared to those with the lowest.[310]

This exciting data regarding the ability of omega-3 PUFAs to reduce adenomas has spawned more recent research in the realm of a disease we have discussed before called familial adenomatous polyposis (FAP). Recall, in FAP there is a genetic defect that contributes to the development of multiple colorectal adenomas, necessitating colectomy in patients to prevent colorectal cancer. Researchers from the UK and Italy recently completed a randomized, placebo-controlled trial in which patients who had undergone prophylactic colectomy for FAP were given EPA or placebo for six months. Those receiving the omega-3 fatty acid supplement demonstrated a statistically significant 22.4% reduction in polyp number compared to the placebo group.[311] This is an impressive result, considering this decrease in polyp count mirrors that which we previously delineated with cyclooxygenase inhibitor treatment for FAP. Moreover, this illustrates a potent anti-microinflammatory activity of omega-3 fatty acids that could potentially impact the lives of patients with familial adenomatous polyposis.

Although no large-scale trial has been published to date assessing the colorectal cancer treatment potential of isolated omega-3 PUFAs, there have been investigations examining the potential synergism between omega-3 fatty acids and traditional colon cancer therapies. In laboratory studies of colorectal cancer cell lines exposed to a typical colon cancer chemotherapeutic agent known as 5-fluorouracil, both DHA and a mixture of DHA and EPA have demonstrated the ability to synergistically augment 5-fluorouracil's apoptotic properties and enhance its ability to inhibit cellular proliferation.[312,313] Moreover, both DHA and EPA have been shown to improve the cytotoxic effects of radiation therapy in colorectal cancer cell lines.[314] This potential coaction between omega-3 fatty acids and traditional therapies for cancer offers promise in cancer management and further solidifies the convincing antimicroinflammatory activity of natural dietary supplements.

The role of omega-3 fatty acids in the prevention and management of cancers beyond colorectal and breast is less well established and generally poorly studied. Nonetheless, the data on the antimicroinflammatory activities of omega-3 PUFAs is compelling, and the efficacy demonstrated in the breast and colon cancer arenas is undeniable. This certainly provides a foundation for further investigation in other tumor lines, particularly where there is solid evidence for a prominent microinflammatory component to the cancer. In any event, the net positive benefit of omega-3 fatty acids in the microinflammatory space, combined with their relatively innocuous profile, make them a strong consideration for acceptance into the antimicroinflammatory armamentarium.

ADDITIONAL ANTIMICROINFLAMMATICS WITH PROMISE

The scientific evidence surrounding the antimicroinflammatory agents we have just discussed is robust and voluminous and certainly has been subjected to the rigorous scrutiny that has placed them in the spotlight as treatments for microinflammation. There are a host of other agents, however, that show promise on the basis of preliminary research, but have not yet attained the evidence base for universal adaptation. We present a few here with what we consider to be long-term promise in the arena of microinflammation management and urge individuals to keep a watchful eye on them as more data emerges concerning their efficacy in preventing cellular and molecular inflammation.

BROMELAIN

Bromelain is an extract derived from the fruit and stem of the pineapple plant and is comprised of a multitude of constituents, mostly enzymes, which are believed to contribute to its different physiological properties. The principal component of bromelain is a protein-digesting, or proteolytic, enzyme that functions to aid the digestive process by breaking down proteins into their amino acid building blocks. Interestingly, bromelain also contains natural substances known as protease inhibitors that block other enzymes from breaking down specific proteins involved in the immune system and even cancer spread. Bromelain is also known to possess a unique nonproteolytic enzyme known as escharase, which is believed to impart wound-healing activities and contains a host of other constituents, including peroxidase, acid phosphatase, and calcium.[314,315]

Pineapples have a long history of use in folk medicine, principally as digestive aids and treatment for macroinflammatory disorders.[316] Bromelain, however, has only been available commercially as a supplement within the last century. Given its historical use as an anti-inflammatory agent, it should come as no surprise that it has been studied in both the oncology and cardiovascular arenas as another agent to battle chronic low-grade microinflammation. We will explore the available data on bromelain's anti-microinflammatory properties and examine its potential as an adjunct to preventing and treating cancer and atherosclerotic coronary artery disease.

Unlike most of the agents we have explored so far, bromelain appears to have a dual effect on the production of microinflammatory mediators. In nonstimulated immune and inflammatory cells, bromelain appears to induce the secretion of IL-1β, IL-6, TNF-α, and IFNγ, thereby enhancing serum levels of these biomarkers![317-319] However, in stimulated monocytes, bromelain administration produces a profound reduction in the same microinflammatory markers, which appears mediated through reduced activity of NF-κB, a common pathway of microinflammatory inhibition that we have seen with other agents. This dual activity may appear contradictory at first, but it highlights a unique ability of bromelain to "turn on" the microinflammatory processes when they are needed for defense and the appropriate inflammatory cell populations are not yet stimulated, and shut them off when they are activated and producing deleterious microinflammatory insult.

Beyond inhibiting cytokines, bromelain appears to decrease the microinflammatory milieu by reducing COX-2 mRNA, which, as we have seen, is exuberantly expressed in many inflammatory pathways.[320] Additionally, the pineapple extract has been shown to reduce inflammatory cell migration into inflamed regions through its ability to interfere with certain cell surface proteins that prevent the adhesion of cells such as leukocytes to local sites of microinflammatory activity.[321] Furthermore, there is biochemical evidence that bromelain specifically inhibits COX-2 expression, corroborating the results previously delineated regarding its ability to reduce COX-2 mRNA.[322]

Bromelain also appears to selectively alter the synthesis of specific prostaglandins—substances we know are intimately tied to microinflammatory pathways. We have seen that prostaglandins generally exist in two groups, proinflammatory and anti-inflammatory. Bromelain has been shown to selectively change the proportion of proinflammatory to anti-inflammatory prostaglandins, shifting the balance to a net anti-inflammatory effect.[314] This potent activity on prostaglandins certainly contributes to the multitude of microinflammation-suppressing activities inherent in the plant-derived extract.

Finally, bromelain appears to function as a signaling agent, which has important implications in multiple clinical arenas. Studies confirm that bromelain upregulates the critical p53 tumor suppressor protein that we now know is integral in the process of cancer cell apoptosis. It performs another important cellular signaling activity by directly inhibiting NF-κB, which we have also discovered is a common pathway through which much microinflammatory activity flows.[323] Finally, bromelain has been shown to positively affect two critical cellular signaling pathways that protect cardiac muscle cells from death during times of oxygen deprivation.[324] As we shall see, these diverse signaling pathways are incorporated into a host of different physiological effects, allowing bromelain to act in various clinical situations.

Bromelain and Cancer

The first anecdotal reports of bromelain in cancer treatment were reported in the 1970s by Gerard and Nieper, who described remarkable remissions of different malignancies, including breast and ovarian, with high-dose administration of bromelain for several weeks.[325,326] Gerard's study not only demonstrated reduced breast cancer masses, but also revealed decreases in metastatic disease. Nieper's investigation further revealed that lower doses of toxic chemotherapy agents could be given in the presence of high-dose bromelain, decreasing the overall toxicity to patients while yielding the same clinical results on tumor suppression. Since the time of these series, more data has emerged suggesting this pineapple extract may exert inhibitory activity on different types of tumors and specific processes that are involved with tumor growth and differentiation.

In the test tube, bromelain appears to inhibit the cellular growth and invasion capabilities of certain tumor cells.[327-329] In stomach cancer cell lines, the extract has been shown to produce significant growth retardation and DNA alteration, leading to arrested cellular proliferation.[327,328] In other investigations, bromelain has been shown to reduce the invasion or metastatic capacity of certain brain cancer cells, although it did not demonstrate any significant effect on growth inhibition in this tumor type.[330] As we have observed with many other agents, this differential effect likely represents physiological activity on specific pathways utilized by some tumors, but not others.

Other studies have demonstrated bromelain's potential for use as an adjunctive cancer therapy based upon its effects on certain hematologic processes. We have discussed the role of fibrin in the atherosclerotic process, which acts much like a glue that helps solidify blood clots, but have yet to delineate its position in the cancer arena. Ample evidence demonstrates that elevated levels of fibrin, usually measured by quantifying its breakdown products, correlate with increased tumor volume, a higher likelihood of tumor progression, and poor survival in patients with multiple different types of cancers.[331-333] Interestingly, fibrin has demonstrated a protective effect on tumors by inhibiting the cytotoxic activity of our defense cells and producing a protective shield around cancer cells that is resistant to our natural protein-digesting enzymes.[334,335] Bromelain has been shown in multiple investigations to be an effective fibrinolytic agent, allowing it to reduce the available amount of circulating fibrin.[336-338] The yet unproven clinical implication here is that the fibrinolytic properties of bromelain may allow it to degrade the protective fibrin shield around tumor cells, making them more vulnerable to our natural defenses and clinically applied therapies.

Another hematologic activity of bromelain that may have potential utility in the oncology, as well as cardiovascular, arena is its ability to alter platelet activity. We extensively described the action of platelets in the evolution of the clinical symptoms of coronary atherosclerosis, but their importance in the interplay between microinflammation and cancer is also well recognized. Investigation has revealed that cancer cells activate platelets and induce platelet aggregation, in a process similar to that seen when the atherosclerotic fibrous cap ruptures during a heart attack.[339] These platelet aggregates are then utilized by cancer cells to form a different type of protective cloak that helps them escape recognition by our immune systems. Further, as cancer cells mature and metastasize, the platelet aggregates appear to promote endothelial cell adhesion and facilitate invasion into adjacent tissues.[340]

Bromelain has clearly demonstrated the ability to reduce platelet aggregation and activation.[341-343] The potential clinical implication, therefore, is that the administration of bromelain may disrupt the platelet aggregates that are encasing cancer cells, making them visible and vulnerable to our natural immune surveillance processes. Further, by inhibiting platelet activity, the ability of tumor cells to adhere to the endothelium and invade nearby tissues is impeded.

There are certainly many unanswered clinical questions surrounding bromelain's potential as an anticancer agent. However, research to date has illuminated some promising features of this novel fruit-derived extract. Its established activity in microinflammatory pathways that are integral to cancer formation, growth, and proliferation provides a solid foundation for further study and offers hope for bromelain as another adjunctive natural therapy in the prevention and treatment of cancer.

Bromelain and Coronary Artery Disease

Based upon the prior discussion of bromelain in cancer, it should be evident that there is potential overlap in this extract's activity in the cardio-vascular disease arena. Platelet activation and thrombus formation via fibrin activity is an integral part of the atherosclerotic cascade, as plaques rupture and produce unstable coronary syndromes such as heart attacks. Brome-lain's ability to inhibit both fibrin and platelet activity certainly gives rise to the potential for this agent as an adjunctive treatment for patients with acute coronary syndromes, and also as a preventive therapy that can inhibit the platelet activity that contributes to microinflammation.

A recently published review of bromelain's activity in cardiovascular disease reveals that it has potential cardioprotective effects, as subjects with oxygen impairment of their heart muscle demonstrated significant improvement in heart muscle recovery when given bromelain compared to controls who did not receive the extract.[344] Two older studies have reported that bromelain administration prevents or minimizes the severity of angina attacks (chest pain) in patients with established atherosclerotic coronary artery disease. Further, a decreased incidence of heart attack was reported in subjects taking bromelain in association with potassium and magnesium.[345] These promising initial studies, in conjunction with bromelain's established antiplatelet and fibrinolytic activity, pave a path toward greater discovery in the pineapple extract's utility in preventing and treating atherosclerotic coronary artery disease.

Prickly Pear Cactus

Perhaps one of the more intriguing plants that seems to demonstrate promise in the microinflammatory arena is *Opuntia ficus-indica*, or the prickly pear cactus. Prickly pear, also known by many as nopal, is a tropical or subtropical plant with origins in South America that now grows wild in arid and semiarid regions worldwide. Prickly pear has been used as an herbal remedy in many countries, but is quite popular in Mexico, where it has been utilized for a host of conditions, including diabetes mellitus, high cholesterol, atherosclerosis, obesity, alcohol-induced hangover, colitis, diarrhea, and benign prostatic hypertrophy.[346,347] Of particular interest is its use in obesity, diabetes mellitus, high cholesterol, and atherosclerosis, as these are obviously at the heart of the microinflammatory discussion. We will explore its use in these diseases and attempt to understand its role at the cellular and molecular level for diseases with a chronic low-grade inflammatory base.

Prickly pear cactus has long been touted as possessing antioxidant activity. The cladodes, or flattened stem regions, of the plant have been analyzed chemically and contain significant amounts of the antioxidant substances vitamin C, vitamin E, glutathione, and carotenoids. Moreover, they hold an abundance of flavonoids and other phenolic compounds, which we have seen are active as antimicroinflammatory agents.[348] The antioxidant properties of the cactus appear to reside in water-soluble polysaccharides (long, repeating sequences of carbohydrates) that reside in the cell walls of the plant. A recent study has shown that the water-soluble polysaccharides extracted from the *Opuntia ficus-indica* plant effectively inhibit superoxide and hydroxyl radicals, thereby providing a potent antioxidant effect.[349] As we have seen, there is an intimate relationship between oxidative processes and microinflammatory pathways, and this objective identification of the prickly pear cactus's ability to neutralize potent oxidants is paramount to explaining its potential health benefits.

The specific antioxidant effects of prickly pear cactus in humans were examined by a group of Italian researchers in the early twenty-first century. In this investigation, prickly pear fruit was compared to vitamin C in a randomized, double-blind, crossover fashion, in which healthy subjects received each substance for two weeks followed by a six-week washout prior to switching. The primary end point was measurement of oxidative stress by standard laboratory surrogates for redox analysis as well as oxidation status of LDL cholesterol molecules. Investigators discovered that consuming prickly pear fruit was associated with a statistically significant improvement compared to baseline and vitamin C supplementation in all oxidative parameters. Moreover, cactus supplementation resulted in a significant reduction in LDL oxidation, again compared to baseline and vitamin C consumption.[350] We have seen the critical importance of LDL oxidation in the atherosclerotic process. Therefore, by reducing this oxidative modification, this study provides preliminary evidence that prickly pear cactus may produce important cardiovascular risk-reducing effects.

Additional analysis of the prickly pear cactus plant properties reveal that it possesses another key component—dietary fiber. According to the American Heart Association, dietary fiber "has been associated with increased diet quality and decreased risk of cardiovascular disease. Soluble or viscous fibers modestly reduce LDL ("bad") cholesterol beyond levels achieved by diet low in saturated and trans fats and cholesterol alone."[351] In a recently reported biochemical evaluation of prickly pear cactus, researchers reported that both the stem and fruit of the plant have high concentrations of dietary fiber, with a significant proportion of it being the soluble fiber that is beneficial in cholesterol reduction. Investigators also revealed that dietary fiber is critical for transportation of the antimicroinflammatory polyphenol compounds, and they found high concentrations of polyphenols within the prickly pear cactus samples they analyzed.[352] The obvious implication is that prickly pear cactus, with its high dietary fiber and polyphenol combination, could produce a powerful combined effect on cardiovascular risk reduction by lowering bad cholesterol levels and attenuating the microinflammatory milieu at the cellular level.

Prickly Pear Cactus and Cancer

Although our discussion thus far has largely focused on prickly pear cactus's antioxidant and antimicroinflammatory properties as they relate to mechanisms of cardiovascular risk reduction, there is some evidence to suggest that nopal may have utility in the oncology arena. In a recently published investigation, researchers assessed the antioxidant capacity and cancer cell toxicity of nine species of prickly pear cactus. The cactus juice was quantified according to flavonoid content and antioxidant capacity and tested against four different cancer cell lines—liver, colon, prostate, and breast. Of the nine juices tested, one known as *rastrero* had the highest antioxidant capacity and was the only one to demonstrate cytotoxic activity against all four cancer lines. The second highest antioxidant capacity was recorded in the *Gavia* species, which demonstrated the greatest potency against colon cancer cells, with a lesser effect on liver and prostate cells, but no effect on breast cancer lines. Other species with intermediate and low degrees of antioxidant capacity still demonstrated variable levels of cytotoxicity on the different cancer cell lines.[353] This preliminary information creates a provocative foundation for additional investigation into the anticancer effects of the prickly pear cactus.

In a different type of cancer investigation, researchers from India assessed the effect of the active pigment component of prickly pear cactus, known as betanin, on the growth of human leukemia cells. We have previously seen that natural pigments can possess significant bioactivities when we discussed the potent antimicroinflammatory properties of curcumin, the pigment component of turmeric. In this study, investigators isolated betanin from the fruit of the *Opuntia ficus-indica* plant and treated a specific leukemia cell line in the laboratory. Betanin produced potent dose-dependent reductions in leukemia cell growth, as well as apoptosis, and loss of mitochondrial membrane integrity.[354] This apoptotic capacity of prickly pear cactus provides further support of its potential as an anticancer agent and can hopefully spawn additional research that will corroborate its efficacy in chemoprevention or cancer therapy.

Prickly Pear Cactus and Cardiovascular Disease

As we highlighted when discussing the mechanisms of action of prickly pear cactus, there appear to be several pathways by which nopal can produce cardiovascular risk reduction. The most obvious mechanism involves its high soluble fiber content, which helps in cholesterol reduction, combined with its ability to reduce LDL oxidation, which traps it in a form that cannot be ingested by macrophages and incorporated into an atherosclerotic plaque. Shapiro and Gong have confirmed prickly pear cactus's ability to improve lipid profiles in patients with high cholesterol.[355] Although no definitive data is available on the plant's ability to retard atherosclerosis, by inhibiting LDL oxidation, the prickly pear cactus could directly confront the microinflammation that is occurring at the endothelial border and inhibit plaque deposition within the arterial walls. Of course, at this point, these cellular effects are merely speculative, and more detailed trials need to be undertaken to better elucidate prickly pear's efficacy in this regard.

Another potential pathway for prickly pear cactus to reduce microinflammation and improve cardiovascular risk is through its apparent ability to control diabetes mellitus. We previously detailed the deleterious effects of impaired glucose tolerance and have clearly established the link between glucose aberrations and the presence of microinflammation. Prickly pear cactus has been used extensively in many Latin American cultures for the treatment of diabetes mellitus, and this anecdotal use is now founded in scientific evidence. In one placebo-controlled crossover study conducted in the 1990s, patients were given broiled prickly pear cactus stems, and glucose levels were monitored post-ingestion. The nopal produced an average glucose reduction of 48 milligrams per deciliter compared to baseline levels.[356] Others have reported similar benefits of prickly pear cactus ingestion, corroborating its efficacy in reducing serum glucose levels.[355,357] These effects, combined with the cactus's potential for improving cholesterol profiles, make it an attractive agent for further research as a natural modulator of cardiovascular risk.

Clearly, there is foundational promise for prickly pear cactus as an adjunctive therapy in the microinflammatory arsenal. The preliminary evidence in both the cancer and cardiovascular arenas is promising, and brings us one step closer to adding yet another natural agent to the list of efficacious compounds in the fight against the untoward effects of microinflammation.

CHAPTER 7: PUTTING IT ALL TOGETHER

Scientific advancement has provided us with evolving insight into the mechanisms of disease and the therapeutic options available for preventing and treating potentially lethal conditions. New technologies have allowed us to better diagnose diseases and even detect them at earlier stages, allowing for more prompt and judicious treatment. Clinical investigation continues to divulge new management paradigms, and an enhanced focus on evidence-based medicine has directed practitioners to adopt more rigorous, scientifically validated treatment plans. With all of these developments, people are living longer and surviving conditions that were fatal many decades ago. Despite this, diseases such as coronary atherosclerosis and cancer remain major killers in the world, taking innumerable lives each year. Indeed, we still have much work to do and must continue to better understand these processes so that we can not only provide superior treatment, but devise more sophisticated prevention strategies to decrease disease prevalence.

Understanding the microinflammatory linkage to these processes is not only a step forward in appreciating the complexity of these conditions, but allows us to create a tangible target for strategies that can be directed toward preventing diseases such as cancer and coronary atherosclerosis. For the past couple of decades, we have focused much on oxidative stress and its adverse effects on our systems, propelling antioxidant therapy to the center of nutritional remedies. Emerging science in microinflammation, however, takes us one step deeper and allows us to better understand that the cellular and biochemical derangements actually result from chronic low-grade inflammation, which, in turn, can instigate oxidative processes. Moreover, we now know that microinflammatory pathways are responsible for the physiological alterations that result in cancer cells having the ability to proliferate unchecked or cholesterol molecules to accumulate within the walls of coronary arteries, and this is a powerful foundation for designing therapies that can arrest, or at least impede, these processes. Ultimately, understanding microinflammation allows us to focus on disease prevention rather than disease treatment.

But primary prevention is a multifaceted process, requiring a concerted effort by both the physician and the patient. The physician is charged with performing an aggressive risk factor assessment and developing a plan for behavioral, dietary, and lifestyle modification, while the patient must commit to risk-reducing actions and therapies. Only by working together can practitioners and patients effectively devise a strategy to prevent disease.

This is seemingly straightforward, but executing a synergistic plan of action between patients and practitioners has its challenges. We have already poignantly described theself destructive nature of obesity and diabetes mellitus, as poor dietary and physical fitness habits have caused these conditions to reach epidemic proportions worldwide. Moreove, the prevalence of these devastating diseases incites the microinflammation that underlies much of coronary disease, cancer, and even premature aging. Most people will readily admit they understand obesity and diabetes are unhealthy precursors to more harmful diseases, yet, as indicated by the increasing prevalence of both conditions, do nothing about it. Why do we ignore our unhealthy lifestyles and continue to engage in behaviors that increase our risk of developing disease? Why do we not readily take ownership in our own preventive health and instead rely on others to tell us what we need to do, even though we largely know exactly what we need to do?

The answers to these questions is likely multifaceted and incorporates several fundamental facts. Principally, obesity and diabetes mellitus generally do not make us feel poorly except when there are acute complications of diabetes or when we become morbidly obese. Most of us also derive great pleasure in eating unhealthy, fat-filled foods, because they simply tend to taste better than healthier alternatives such as raw vegetables and oatmeal. Further, regular exercise takes time and often discomfort at some level, particularly for those of us already used to a sedentary lifestyle. As a result, the path of least resistance leads us to poor dietary habits and inactivity—the necessary ingredients to create obesity and diabetes.

But patients aren't solely to blame, as we have already indicated that prevention has largely been a secondary goal of traditional medical practitioners. Conventional medical education has always focused on diagnosing and treating diseases, and only in recent decades has primary prevention held more of the spotlight. Despite this more recent emphasis on preventive medicine, however, many practitioners continue to prioritize diagnosis and treatment. Moreover, many practitioners, whether due to time constraints or simply lack of interest, do not regularly follow the primary prevention literature, or wait for primary prevention strategies to be published in practice guidelines (which may be many years after they have been scientifically validated). Furthermore, physicians are often reticent to adopt new technologies or incorporate new ideas into their practices unless such changes meet specific, often personally derived standards. On top of all this, there is considerable variability in the degree to which practitioners believe in the diverse facets of primary prevention, and even greater aberration in their understanding of the role that nonprescription nutraceutical agents play in preventing disease.

So we, practitioners and patients alike, must take ownership of the wealth of data that is out there, decide how we fit into a particular risk pool, and determine which strategies for prevention will have the greatest benefit and lowest risk. By no means is this an easy task, but utilizing the microinflammatory arena as a foundation, there are several steps that can be taken to assure that patients and practitioners are truly doing all they can for disease prevention.

First of all, practitioners and patients must objectively look at one another and address the modifiable risk factors that truly form the foundation of microinflammatory insult. Physicians must objectively measure a patient's height, weight, and abdominal circumference like any other vital sign and speak candidly about the risk that accompanies even a small elevation in body mass index. Patients must look in the mirror and take no insult from a discussion of weight loss, understanding the first step toward fighting obesity is admitting that it exists. By emphasizing the overwhelming health benefits of obesity reduction, both practitioner and patient alike can develop a goal-directed plan to reduce this overly prevalent and readily modifiable risk factor.

And by attacking this one risk, it must be emphasized that there could be a concomitant elimination of at least two other important and modifiable risk factors: diabetes mellitus and high cholesterol As we have described, diabetes mellitus is largely a byproduct of the obesity epidemic, as the microinflammatory insult of corpulence produces insulin resistance, the defining characteristic of type 2 diabetes. Moreover, the obesity-induced microinflammation of the liver contributes to elevated LDL cholesterol levels that increase the pool of available lipid molecules that can be oxidized and incorporated into growing atherosclerotic plaques. By aggressively treating obesity, the microinflammatory state can be dramatically attenuated, and diseases such as hypercholesterolemia and diabetes mellitus may actually disappear. Moreover, by reducing the microinflammatory environment and diminishing or eliminating these risk factors, we have shown that the processes of coronary atherosclerosis, cancer formation, and even premature aging can be decelerated or event arrested. Modification of this epidemic risk factor can truly produce amazing changes to an individual's health profile!

Aside from presenting the benefits of aggressive obesity management and stringent diabetes control, we have illustrated the utility of advanced risk screening assessments that can add prognostic information to our baseline patient risk analyses. For example, incorporating the readily available inflammatory biomarkers hs-CRP and Lp-PLA$_2$ into our risk stratification paradigm, we can identify an even greater proportion of the population at risk for cardiovascular events and more aggressively treat them with a primary prevention regimen. Moreover, it is clear that continued evolution in the genetics of disease will soon allow us to incorporatecertain genetic testing into our prevention armamentarium. Cancer research is probably furthest along in this arena, as many genetic tests are currently in use to risk-stratify patients and even personalize tumor therapy. Along these same lines, we may soon be able to utilize SIRT1 gene analysis or telomere length measurements as a marker to predict risk or response to treatment.

Moving from risk assessment to aggressive risk intervention, we have presented a wealth of information on a variety of prescription and non-prescription compounds that are effective in suppressing microinflammation, and it is worthwhile to discuss some of the clinical synergy that can be derived from specific agents. We detailed the immense data on aspirin's chemopreventive properties, and most individuals are familiar with the clinical protection that this time-tested medication provides against stroke, heart attack, and other manifestations of cardiac and vascular disease. Individuals who are already candidates for aspirin therapy based upon preexisting clinical conditions obviously benefit not only from its primary activity in those diseases, but also gain its antimicroinflammatory and pharmacopreventive attributes. Similar synergism may be derived for individuals with diabetes mellitus or polycystic ovary disease who take metformin, those with peripheral vascular disease who take pentoxifylline, those with high cholesterol who take statins, and those with arthritis who take COX-2 inhibitors. The multi-facetedbenefits of these and other medicines can be powerful and certainly need to be considered in a risk-benefit analysis for primary prevention. Again, this is a discussion that must take place with an appropriate health-care provider well versed in the prevention arena.

Exploring the antimicroinflammatory arena even further, we have provided a substantive, but not exhaustive appraisal of a multitude of other agents that demonstrate great promise in attenuating the microinflammation that resides at the foundation of many diseases. We illustrated that simple, often overlooked trace elements such as zinc, magnesium, and selenium can have powerful effects in modulating microinflammatory processes and that even in the United States, many people do not meet their daily requirements of such important minerals. Further, we detailed the significance of vitamin D and E as microinflammatory mitigators, highlighting their potent effects in cancer and cardiovascular disease, respectively. With a little education, individuals can take ownership of ensuring compliance with at least minimal recommended daily allowances of these trace elements and derive at least some benefit from their microinflammation-fighting properties. Moreover, this is one arena that can largely be addressed without input from health-care providers. Having said that, it is important for all individuals to understand that supplements of any kind can have important interactions with many prescription and nonprescription medicines, so caution must be exercised by those already taking medications before venturing into a supplement regimen. Additionally, it is important to avoid the "more is better" philosophy with regard to nutraceuticals, as excess ingestion of vitamins, minerals, and other supplements can have potentially harmful and counterproductive effects.

Beyond trace elements, we provided a detailed discussion of myriad natural substances that have years of extensive study behind them, and explained the science and potential of agents that have long histories of therapeutic use in folk medicine. The prospective benefits of resveratrol, omega-3 fatty acids, quercetin, and curcumin cannot be denied, and the emerging science behind agents such as bromelain and prickly pear cactus is exciting and adds new promise to the investigational arena for primary prevention.

At the end of the day, aggressive risk factor assessment and treatment really establishes the foundation for primary prevention. Utilizing traditional risk assessment by measuring cholesterol levels, blood pressure, height, weight, glucose, etc. is an important part of health screening for anyone, but it doesn't stop there. We have more sophisticated markers, such as CRP and Lp-PLA$_2$, that allow us to better understand the microinflammatory risk that we now know propagates cancer, coronary disease, and aging. By better identifying individuals at risk, implementing aggressive strategies to reduce it, and keeping an open mind about adjunctive therapeutic options, we, as practitioners and patients, can more effectively battle the potentially lethal microinflammation that characterizes two of the most lethal diseases in the world, and the process of aging itself.

GLOSSARY

adenoma: A general term that refers to any benign tumor that originates from a gland. Polyps in the colon are a type of adenoma, but they may be present in any number of tissues or organs throughout the body. Many adenomas have the potential to become malignant over time and transform into cancers.

adipocytes: Fat cells.

adipokines: Proteins that are produced and secreted by fat cells that signal other cells or tissues to perform specific functions.

advanced glycation end products (AGEs): The result of a chemical interaction between a sugar molecule and a protein or lipid that results in a relatively permanent bond between them. AGEs mediate some of the adverse cellular effects of diabetes mellitus.

anaphase: The fourth phase of mitosis, which is marked by complete separation of the chromosomes as they migrate to opposite poles of the cell.

apolipoproteins: A group of proteins that function to bind and carry fats and cholesterol in the blood stream.

apoptosis: A process also known as programmed cell death, whereby defects in a cell or other signals trigger it to self-destruct.

atherosclerosis: The process of cholesterol accumulating in the walls of an artery to form a plaque. This is the fundamental process that leads to heart attacks, strokes, and symptoms of peripheral artery disease (PAD).

body mass index (BMI): A measurement that is used to characterize a patient's obesity status. It is calculated by dividing an individual's weight in kilograms by his/her height in meters squared.

C-reactive protein (CRP): One of the acute phase proteins that is liberated by the liver in response to inflammation and serves as a chemical marker for the microinflammatory process.

carcinogen: Any agent that is directly implicated in causing cancer. This includes chemicals, tobacco, radiation, some viruses, and many other agents.

carcinogenesis: The process of cancer cell formation. Also known as oncogenesis or tumorigenesis.

cell cycle: The process whereby a cell divides and replicates. It consists of four phases, known as G_1, S, G_2, and M. The G_1 and G_2 phases involve cellular growth, S phase is marked by DNA synthesis, and M phase involves mitosis.

centromere: The region of the chromosome that forms the attachment point for sister chromatids as well as the spindle fibers. The spindle fibers are attached to the centromere via the protein constituents known as kinetochores.

chromatid: Refers to one of two identical copies of replicated DNA from an intact chromosome that is joined to its counterpart by a centromere. Most commonly, the chromatid pair are denoted as sister chromatids.

chromosome: An aggregate of DNA and associated proteins coiled into a specific configuration containing multiple genes and functions to house an organism's genetic information.

cyclooxygenase (COX): An enzyme that is directly involved in the inflammatory process by specifically creating prostaglandins from the omega-6 polyunsaturated fatty acid arachidonic acid. Two COX enzymes, COX-1 and COX-2, are principally involved in the microinflammatory pathways.

cytokines: Proteins that are produced by various cells in the body that have important signaling properties and also function as biomarkers of the microinflammatory process.

cytokinesis: The final stage of cell division that occurs following mitosis where cellular cytoplasm is formed and divided, resulting in the formation of two identical replicas of the original cell.

cytoplasm: Refers to the substance within a cell that resides outside of the nucleus, but within the cell membrane. The cytoplasm contains important constituents like mitochondria and is the place where most cellular activities occur.

diastolic blood pressure: The lowest pressure exerted in the arteries when the heart is relaxed. This is expressed as the bottom number in a blood pressure reading.

double-blind study: A research investigation in which neither the investigator nor the subject know whether or not the subject is receiving active or placebo treatment.

endothelial dysfunction: An abnormal state in which the innermost lining of the walls of blood vessels known as the endothelium does not carry out its normal functions of regulating blood vessel constriction and dilatation, mediating aspects of blood clotting, and modulating immune function.

endothelium: The single cell layer that lines the inner surface of blood vessels. Endothelial cells have important regulatory functions in blood vessels and are active in the atherosclerotic process.

erythrocyte sedimentation rate(ESR): A blood test commonly used to determine whether or not there is active inflammation in an individual.

familial adenomatous polyposis: An inherited condition characterized by the formation of numerous colon polyps in affected individuals. Affected subjects are at high risk for developing colon cancer.

fibrinogen: A protein involved in the coagulation cascade that is produced by the liver and converted into fibrin to form a mesh-like network during blood clotting. Fibrinogen is another acute phase reactant that is produced in response to inflammatory stimuli.

free radicals: An atom or group of atoms that possess unpaired electrons. These molecules are highly reactive and are responsible for the damaging cellular effects that occur as a result of oxidative stress.

gene expression: The process by which information encoded on a gene is used to create a protein end product that can be used for physiological processes.

gene transcription, or transcription: The initial process of gene expression in which a segment of DNA is copied into a complementary strand of RNA.

gene translation, or translation: The stage of gene expression in which the RNA strand created during transcription is decoded to produce a strand of amino acids that will ultimately become the desired protein molecule.

hepatocyte: A liver cell.

high-density lipoprotein (HDL): Also designated as HDL cholesterol, this is the "good cholesterol" that is responsible for transporting cholesterol particles out of the bloodstream and back to the liver. Healthcare providers generally try to raise a patient's HDL cholesterol to high levels.

hypertrophy: The process of a cell increasing in size, usually resulting in enlargement of the tissue or organ that is comprised of those cells. A common example is heart muscle hypertrophy that usually occurs with high blood pressure.

interferons: Specific cytokines that are produced and released largely in response to immune activation or the presence of tumor cells. They are responsible for activating immune cells in response to infections and have a pivotal role in stimulating p53 activity. A common interferon is interferon alpha (IFN-α).

interleukins: Specific cytokines that are principally produced by immune cells that are active in immune and inflammatory signaling processes. Common examples include IL-1, IL-6, and IL-1β, and these can be utilized as biomarkers of microinflammation.

interphase: Refers to the portion of the cell cycle that incorporates the G_1, S, and G_2 phases. This is where a cell prepares for division by increasing in size and replicating its DNA so that it can enter mitosis and form two identical daughter cells.

kinetochore: Protein molecules that are used to attach spindle fibers to the chromatids during mitosis.

lipoprotien-associated phospholipase A2 (Lp-PLA2): An enzyme that works preferentially to cleave oxidized phospholipids, such as those found in oxidized LDL particles, that is avidly expressed in atherosclerotic plaques and can serve as a microinflammatory biomarker. Elevated serum levels of Lp-PLA$_2$ correlate with increased risk for cardiac events and stroke.

low-density lipoprotein (LDL): Also designated as LDL cholesterol, this is the "bad cholesterol" that, when oxidized, gets incorporated into an atherosclerotic plaque. Health-care providers generally try to lower LDL to specific targets that are known to protect against atherosclerotic plaque development.

macrophage: A specific type of white blood cell that functions as a scavenger, enveloping other molecules, including cells, bacteria, debris, and cholesterol. Macrophages have a critical role in the atherosclerotic process and are key inflammatory and immune cells.

matrix metalloproteinase: An enzyme that requires the use of a metal, usually zinc, that possesses the ability to break down extracellular proteins. They are important in breaking down the fibrous cap that surrounds an atherosclerotic plaque.

metaphase: The third phase of mitosis, characterized by the alignment of the chromosomes along the metaphase plate that begin to be pulled apart by the spindle apparatus.

mitochondria: The energy-producing factories of a cell.

mitosis: The process of cell division during which the cell divides the DNA replicated in prior steps, and other cellular contents, in half to form two identical copies of the original cell.

monocyte: A specific type of white blood cell that is actually a precursor to the macrophage and functions as an immune and inflammatory mediator.

nuclear factor kappa B (NF-κB): A critical protein that is integral to many microinflammatory pathways, which primarily functions in controlling DNA transcription. NF-κB activation occurs in response to numerous microinflammatory stimuli, including TNF-α, IL-1β, and even reactive oxygen species.

nucleus: The membrane-enclosed region of a cell that houses all of the DNA material in the form of chromosomes.

oncogenesis: See *carcinogenesis*.

oxidant: A chemical or substance also known as an oxidizing agent that removes electrons from another reactant in a chemical reaction. Through this process, the oxidant becomes reduced, and the other reactant becomes oxidized.

oxidative stress: A process also known as redox imbalance in which there is a relative excess of oxidants that can produce damage to specific cellular components such as DNA, proteins, and membranes.

p53 gene: A gene tlocated on chromosome 17 in the human genome that codes for the p53 protein important in preventing cancer.

p53 protein: A protein produced by the p53 gene, also known as tumor suppressor p53, or tumor protein 53, that is involved in regulating the cell cycle and preventing cancer cell transformation.

phagocyte: A general term used for a type of cell that has the capability to engulf other cells, debris, or other particulate matter.

placebo: A term generally applied to a treatment that is given in a research study that has no known medical effect. This allows a baseline against which researchers can compare the effects of an experimental treatment.

placebo-controlled study: A type of research study that involves comparing the effect of an experimental agent with a potential therapeutic effect against an agent that has no known therapeutic effect.

prometaphase: The second stage of mitosis, characterized by the chromosomes forming protein constituents known as kinetochores, which will attach to kinetochore microtubules that stretch from one centrosome to the other on opposite poles of the cell. Prometaphase ends as the microtubules begin to shift the chromosomes to the center of the cell.

prophase: The first phase of mitosis, during which the nuclear DNA consolidates into coiled pieces of DNA known as chromosomes. Additionally, structural components known as centrosomes begin to migrate to opposite poles of the cell and begin to set up a network of cylindrical fibers known as microtubules that will be used to mechanically pull the cell apart.

randomized study: A type of research study in which patients are randomly assigned to one treatment regimen or another. Oftentimes patients are randomized to receive active treatment versus placebo.

Ras protein: Intracellular signaling molecules that are responsible for promoting appropriate cell growth and differentiation. Overactive Ras proteins can stimulate cancer growth.

reactive oxygen species (ROS): Highly reactive molecules that are produced as byproducts of metabolism, contain oxygen, and function as oxidants in oxidation-reduction reactions. An increase in reactive oxygen species characterizes the oxidative stress state.

receptor for advanced glycation end products: A cell membrane receptor that is able to bind advanced glycation end products (AGEs), resulting in the activation of proinflammatory genes.

redox state: Refers to relative balance between oxidized and reduced substances present in a physiological system.

senescence: The process of aging.

sirtuin 1 (SIRT1): The human enzyme encoded by the SIRT1 gene that may be involved in antiaging processes.

systolic blood pressure: The maximum amount of pressure exerted in the arteries during contraction of the heart. This is expressed as the top number in a blood pressure reading.

telophase: The final phase of mitosis, during which the remnant nuclear material of the parent cell envelops each of the daughter cells, thereby creating a new nucleus for each of the daughters.

triglycerides: A type of circulating animal or vegetable fat in the blood that functions as an energy source for many bodily tissues. Elevated triglyceride levels, however, increase the risk for developing cardiovascular disease.

tumor necrosis factors: A specific group of cytokines, principally secreted by monocytes, that are responsible for triggering apoptosis and inducing cellular death. The most active tumor necrosis factor is tumor necrosis factor alpha (TNF-α).

tumorigenesis: See *carcinogenesis*.

NOTES

Chapter 1: The Harsh Reality

1. Hoyert D, Xu J. (2012). Deaths: Preliminary Data for 2011. *National Vital Statistics Reports*, volume 61.

2. "The Top 10 Causes of Death." *WHO*. World Health Organization, n.d. Web. 13 Jan. 2013. <http://www.who.int/mediacentre/factsheets/fs310/en/index.html>.

Chapter 2: Understanding Oxidative Stress

1. Finkel T. (1999). Signal transduction by reactive oxygen species in non-phagocytic cells. *Journal of Leukocyte Biology*, volume 65, 337-340.

2. Shah A, Channon K. (2004). Free radicals and redox signaling in cardiovascular disease. *Heart*, volume 90, 485-487.

3. Li J, Shah A. (2004). Endothelial cell superoxide generation: regulation and relevance for cardiovascular physiology. *American Journal of Physiology*, volume 287, R1014-R1030.

4. Trush M. (1991). An overview of the relationship between oxidative stress and chemical carcinogenesis. *Free Radical Biology and Medicine*, volume 10, 201-209.

5. Barber D. (1994). Oxygen free radicals and antioxidants: a review. *Am Pharm*, volume 34, 26-35.

6. Halliwell B. (1996). Mechanisms involved in the generation of free radicals. *Pathological Biology*, volume 44, 6-13.

7. Kerr L, et al. (1992). Signal transduction: the nuclear target. *Current Opinion in Cell Biology*, volume 4, 496-501.

8. Schenk H. (1994). Distinct effects of thioredoxin and antioxidants on the activation of transcription factors NF-κB and AP-1. *Proceedings of the National Academy of Sciences USA*, volume 91, 1672-1676.

9. Vogelstein B. (2000). Surging the p53 network. *Nature*, volume 408, 307-310.

10. Harris SL, Levine AJ. (2005). The p58 pathway: positive and negative feedback loops. *Oncogene*, volume 24, 2899-2908.

11. Karin M, et al. (1997). AP-1 function and regulation. *Current Opinion in Cell Biology*, volume 9, 240-246.

12. Piette J, et al. (1997). Multiple redox regulation in NF-κB transcription factor activation. *Biological Chemistry*, volume 378, 1237-1245.

13. Valori C, et al. (1967). Free noradrenaline and adrenaline excretion in relation to clinical syndromes following myocardial infarction. *American Journal of Cardiology*, volume 20, 605-617.

14. Francis G, et al. (1982). Relationship of exercise capacity to resting left ventricular performance and basal plasma norepinephrine levels in patients with congestive heart failure. *American Heart Journal*, volume 104, 725-731.

15. Singal P, et al. (1983). Potential oxidative pathways of catecholamines in the formation of lipid peroxides and genesis of heart disease. *Advances in Experimental Medicine and Biology*, volume 161, 391-401.

16. Bernier M, et al. (1989). Reperfusion arrhythmias: dose-related protection by anti-free radical interventions. *American Journal of Physiology*, volume 256, H1344-H1352.

17. Beresewicz A, Horackova M. (1991). Alterations in electrical and contractile behavior of isolated cardiomyocytes by hydrogen peroxide: possible ionic mechanisms. *Journal of Molecular and Cellular Cardiology*, volume 23, 899-918.

18. Witztum J, Steinberg D. (1991). Role of oxidized low-density lipoprotein in atherogenesis. *Journal of Clinical Investigation*, volume 88, 1785-1792.

19. Harman D. (1956). Aging: a theory base on free radical and radiation chemisty. *Journal of Gerontology*, volume 11, 298-300.

20. Harman D. (1972). The biologic clock: the mitochondria? *Journal of the American Geriatric Society*, volume 20, 145-147.

21. Miguel J, et al. (1980). Mitochondrial role in cell aging. *Experimental Gerontology*, volume 15, 575-591.

22. Ames B, et al. (1993). Oxidants, antioxidants, and the degenerative diseases of aging. *Proceedings of the National Academy of Sciences USA*, volume 90, 917, 915-922.

23. Stadtman E. (1992). Protein oxidation and aging. *Science*, volume 257, 1220-1224.

24. Berlett BS, Stadtman ER. (1997). Protein oxidation in aging, disease, and oxidative stress. *Journal of Biological Chemistry*, volume 272, 20313-20316.

25. Beckman K, Ames B. (1998). The free radical theory of aging matures. *Physiological Reviews*, volume 78, 547-581.

26. Beckman K. (1998). Mitochondrial aging: open questions. *Annals of the New York Academy of Science*, volume 854, 118-127.

27. Sohal R, et al. (1995). Mitochondrial superoxide and hydrogen peroxide generation, protein oxidative damage, and longevity in different species of flies. *Free Radical Biology and Medicine*, volume 19(4), 499-504.

28. Sohal R, Weindruch R. (1996) Oxidative Stress, Caloric Restriction, and Aging. *Science*, volume 273 (5271), 59-63.

29. Esser K, Martin G. (1995). *Molecular Aspects of Aging*. Chichester: J. Wiley and Sons.

30. Sen C, et al. (2000) *Handbook of Oxidants and Antioxidants in Exercise*. Elsevier Science B.V., Amsterdam.

31. McCay C, et al. (1935). The effect of retarded growth upon the length of life span and upon the ultimate body size. *Journal of Nutrition*, volume 35, 63-79.

32. Yu B, et al. (1982). Life span study of SPF Fischer 344 male rates fed ad libitum or restricted diets: longevity, growth, lean body mass and disease. *Journal of Gerontology*, volume 37, 130-141.

33. Houthoofd K, Vanfetern J. (2006). Longevity effect of dietary restriction in *Caenorhabditis elegans*. *Experimental Gerontology*, volume 41, 1026-1032.

34. Colman R, et al. (2009). Caloric restriction delays disease onset and mortality in rhesus monkeys. *Science*, volume 325, 201-204.

35. Tolmasoff J, et al. (1980). Superoxide dismutase: correlation with life-span and specific metabolic rate in primate species. *Proceedings of the National Academy of Sciences USA*, volume 77, 2777-2781.

36. Muller-Hocker J. (1989). Cytochrome c oxidase deficient cardiomyocytes in the human heart—an age-related phenomenon: a histochemical ultracytochemical study. *American Journal of Pathology*, volume 134, 1167-1173.

37. Muller-Hocker J. et al. (1993). Different in situ hydridization patterns of mitochondrial DNA in cytochrome c oxidase-deficient extraocular muscle fibers in the elderly. *Virchows Archiv*, volume 422, 7-15.

38. Trounce I, et al. (1989). Decline in skeletal muscle mitochondrial respiratory chain function: possible factor in ageing. *Lancet*, volume 1, 637-639.

39. Lesnefsky E, Hoppel C. (2006). Oxidative phosphorylation and aging. *Ageing Research Reviews*, volume 5, 402-433.

40. Hayakawa M, et al. (1991). Age-associated accumulation of 8-hydroxydeoxygquanosine in mitochondrial DNA of human diaphragm. *Biochemical and Biophysical Research Communications*, volume 179, 1023-1029.

41. Hayahawa M, et al. (1992). Age-associated oxygen damage and mutations in mitochondrial DNA in human heart. *Biochemical and Biophysical Research Communications*, volume 189, 979-985.

42. Liu C, et al. (2004). Mitochondrial DNA mutation and depletion increase the susceptibility of human cells to apoptosis. *Annals of the New York Academy of Science*, volume 1011, 133-145.

43. Taylor R, Turnbull D. (2005). Mitochondrial DNA mutations in human disease. *Nature Reviews Genetics*, volume 6, 389-402.

44. Higami Y, Shimokawa I. (2000). Apoptosis in the aging process. *Cell Tissue Research*, volume 301, 125-132.

45. Singal, P, et al. (1998). The role of oxidative stress in the genesis of heart disease. *Cardiovascular Research*, volume 40, 426-432.

46. Lin M, Beal M. (2006). Mitochondrial dysfunction and oxidative stress in neurodegenerative diseases. *Nature*, volume 443, 787-795.

47. Giordano F. (2005). Oxygen, oxidative stress, hypoxia and heart failure. *Journal of Clinical Investigation*, volume 115, 500-508.

48. Cave A. (2005). NADPH oxidase-derived reactive oxygen species in cardiac pathophysiology. *Philosophical Transactions of the Royal Society*, volume 360, 2327-2334.

49. Gao W, et al. (1996). Selective effects of oxygen free radicals on excitation-contraction coupling in ventricular muscle: implications for the mechanism of stunned myocardium. *Circulation*, volume 94, 2597-2604.

50. Ide T, et al. (2001). Mitochondrial DNA damage and dysfunction associate with oxidative stress in failing hearts after myocardial infarction. *Circulation Research*, volume 88, 529-535.

51. Doroshow, J. (1983). Effect of anthracycline antibiotics on oxygen radical formation in rat heart. *Cancer Research*, volume 43, 460-472.

52. Singal, P, Iliskovis N. (1998). Doxorubicin-induced cardiomyopathy. *New England Journal of Medicine*, volume 339(13), 900-905.

53. Siveski-Iliskovic N. (1995). Probucol protects against Adriamycin cardiomyopathy without interfering with its antitumor effect. *Circulation*, volume 91, 10-15.

54. Myers C, et al. (1977). Adriamycin: the role of lipid peroxidation in cardiac toxicity and tumor response. *Science*, volume 19, 165-167.

55. Guyton K, Kensler T. (1993). Oxidative mechanisms in carcinogenesis. *British Medical Bulletin*, volume 49, 523-544.

56. Schulte-Herman R, et al. (1990). DNA synthesis, apoptosis, and phenotypic expression as determinants of growth of altered foci in rat liver during phenobarbital promotion. *Cancer Research*, volume 50, 5127-5135.

57. Klaunig J, et al. (1998). The role of oxidative stress in chemical cardinogenesis. *Environmental Health Perspectives*, volume 106(suppl 1), 289-295.

58. Frenkel K. (1992). Carcinogen-mediated oxidant formation and oxidative DNA damage. *Pharmacology and Therapeutics*, volume 53, 127-166.

59. Shacter E, et al. (1988). Activated neutrophils induced prolonged DNA damage in neighboring cells. *Carcinogenesis*, volume 9, 2297-2304.

60. Storz P. (2005). Reactive oxygen species in tumor progression. *Frontiers of Bioscience*, volume 10, 1881-1896.

61. Trush, M. (1991). An overview of the relationship between oxidative stress and chemical carcinogenesis. *Free Radical Biology and Medicine*, volume 10, 201-209.

62. Cerutti, P. (1985). Inflammation and oxidative stress in carcinogenesis. *Cancer Cells*, volume 3, 1-7.

63. Muller J, et al. (1997). Antioxidants as well as oxidants activate c-fos via Ras-dependent activity of extracellular signal-regulated kinase 2 and Elk-1. *European Journal of Biochemistry*, volume 244, 45-52.

64. Pennington, J, et al. (2005). Redox-senstive signaling factors as novel molecular targets for cancer therapy, *Drug Resistance Updates*, volume 8, 322-330.

Chapter 3: Microinflammation

1. Libby, P, et al. (2009). Inflammation in atherosclerosis: from patho-physiology to practice. *Journal of the American College of Cardiology*, volume 54, 2129-2138.

2. Trogan E, et al. (2006). Gene expression changes in foam cells and the role of chemokine receptor CCR7 during atherosclerosis regression in ApoE-deficient mice. *Proceedings of the National Academy of Sciences USA*, volume 103, 3781-3786.

3. Van Gils, J, et al. (2012). The neuroimmune guidance cue netrin-1 promotes atherosclerosis by inhibiting the emigration of macrophages from plaques. *Nature Immunology*, volume 13, 136-143.

4. Lippy, P, Aikawa M. (2002). Stabilization of atherosclerotic plaques: new mechanisms and clinical targets. *Nature Medicine*, volume 8, 1257-1262.

5. Mizuno, Y, et al. (2011). Inflammation and the development of athero-sclerosis—effects of lipid-lowering therapy. *Journal of Athersclerosis and Thrombosis*, volume 18, 351-358.

6. Naruko, T, et al. (2002). Neutrophil infiltration of culprit lesions in acute coronary syndromes. *Circulation*, volume 106, 2894-2900.

7. Lindhal B, et al. (2000). Markers of myocardial damage and inflam-mation in relation to long-term mortality in unstable coronary artery disease. *New England Journal of Medicine*, volume 343, 1139-1147.

8. Ridker P, et al. (2000). Plasma concentration of interleukin-6 and the risk of future myocardial infarction among apparently healthy men. *Circulation*, volume 101, 1767-1772.

9. Rader D. (2000). Inflammatory markers of coronary risk. *New England Journal of Medicine*, volume 343, 1179-1182.

10. Ridker P. (2007). C-reactive protein and the prediction of cardiovascular events among those at intermediate risk: moving an inflammatory hypothesis toward consensus. *Journal of the American College of Cardiology*, volume 49, 2129-2138.

11. Ridker P. (2007). Development and validation of improved algorithms for the assessment of global cardiovascular risk in women: the Reynolds Risk Score. *Journal of the American Medical Association*, volume 297, 611-619.

12. Ridker P, et al. (1999). Long-term effects of pravastatin on plasma concentration of C-reactive protein. The Cholesterol and Recurrent Events (CARE) Investigators. *Circulation*, volume 100, 230-235.

13. Ridker P, et al. (2005). Relative efficacy of atorvastatin 80 mg and pravastatin 40 mg in achieving the dual goals of low-density lipoprotein cholesterol < 70 mg/dl and C-reactive protein < 2 mg/l: an analysis of the PROVE IT TIMI-22 trial. *Journal of the American College of Cardiology*, volume 45, 1644-1648.

14. Morrow D, et al. (2006). Clinical relevance of C-reactive protein during follow-up of patients with acute coronary syndromes in the Aggrastat-to-Zocor Trial. *Circulation*, volume 114, 281-288.

15. Ridker P, et al. (2001). Measurement of C-reactive protein for the targeting of statin therapy in the primary prevention of acute coronary events. *New England Journal of Medicine*, volume 344, 1959-1965.

16. Ridker P, et al. (2008). Rosuvastatin to prevent vascular events in men and women with elevated C-reactive protein. *New England Journal of Medicine*, volume 359, 2195-2207.

17. Six D, Dennis E. (2000). The expanding superfamily of phospholipase A(2) enzymes: classification and characterization. *Biochimica et Biophysica Acta*, volume 1488, 1-19.

18. Hakkinen T, et al. (1999). Lipoprotein-associated phospholipase A(2), platelet-activating factor acetylhydrolase, is expressed by macrophages in human and rabbit atherosclerotic lesions. *Arteriosclerosis, Thrombosis, and Vascular Biology*, volume 19, 2909-2917.

19. Krishnankutty S. (2006). Lipoprotein-associated phospholipase A_2, vascular inflammation and cardiovascular risk prediction. *Vascular Health and Risk Management*, volume 2, 153-156.

20. Caslake M, et al. (2000). Lipoprotein-associated phospholipase A(2), platelet-activating factor acetylhydrolase: a potential new risk factor for coronary artery disease. *Atherosclerosis*, volume 150, 413-419.

21. MacPhee C, et al. (1999). Lipoprotein-associated phospholipase A(2), platelet-activating factor acetylhydrolase, generates two bioactive products during the oxidation of low-density lipoprotein: use of a novel inhibitor. *Biochemical Journal*, volume 338, 479-487.

22. Packard C, et al. (2000). Lipoprotein-associated phospholipase A2 as an independent predictor of coronary heart disease. West of Scotland Coronary Prevention Study Group. *New England Journal of Medicine*, volume 343, 1148-1155.

23. Ballantyne C, et al. (2004). Lipoprotein-associated phospholipase A2, high-sensitivity C-reactive protein, and risk of incident coronary heart disease in middle-aged men and women in the Atherosclerosis Risk in Communities (ARIC) study. *Circulation*, volume 109, 837-842.

24. Koenig W, et al. (2004). Lipoprotein-associated phospholipase A2 adds to risk prediction of incident coronary events by C-reactive protein in apparently healthy middle-aged men from the general population: results from the 14-year follow-up of a large cohort from southern Germany. *Circulation*, volume 110, 1903-1908.

25. Oie H, et al. (2005). Lipoprotein-associated phospholipase A2 is associated with risk of coronary heart disease and stroke. The Rotterdam Study. *Circulation*, volume 111, 570-575.

26. Munkhom P. (2003). The incidence and prevalence of colorectal cancer in inflammatory bowel disease. *Alimentary Pharmacology and Therapeutics*, volume 18, 1-5.

27. Lowenfels A, et al. (1993). Pancreatitis and the risk of pancreatic cancer. *New England Journal of Medicine*, volume 328, 1433-1437.

28. Schiffman M, et al. (2007). Human papillomavirus and cervical cancer. *Lancet*, volume 370, 890-907.

29. Watson M, et al. (2008). Using population-based cancer registry data to assess the burden of human papillomavirus-associated cancers in the United States: overview of methods. *Cancer*, volume 113 (suppl 10), 2841-2854.

30. Chaturvedi A, et al. (2011). Human papillomavirus and rising oropharyngeal cancer incidence in the United States. *Journal of Clinical Oncology*, volume 29(32), 4294-4301.

31. Mantovani A. (2009). Cancer: inflaming metastasis. *Nature*, volume 457, 36-37.

32. Hanahan D, Weinberg R. (2000). The hallmarks of cancer. *Cell*, volume 100, 47-70.

33. Hussain S, Harris, C. (2007). Inflammation and cancer: an ancient link with novel potentials. *International Journal of Cancer*, volume 121, 2373-2380.

34. Mantovani A, et al. (2008). Cancer-related inflammation. *Nature*, volume 454, 436-444.

35. Naugler E, Karin, M. (2008). The wolf in sheep's clothing: the role of interleukin-6 in immunity, inflammation and cancer. *Trends in Molecular Medicine*, volume 14, 109-119.

36. Chung Y, Chang Y. (2003). Serum interleukin-6 levels reflect the disease status of colorectal cancer. *Journal of Surgical Oncology*, volume 83, 222-226.

37. Lutgendorf S, et al. (2008). Interleukin-6, cortisol, and depressive symptoms in ovarian cancer patients. *Journal of Clinical Oncology*, volume 26, 4820-4827.

38. Stark J, et al. Circulating prediagnostic interleukin-6 and C-reacitve protein and prostate cancer incidence and mortality. *International Journal of Cancer*, volume 124, 2683-2689.

39. Balkwill F. (2012). Cancer-related inflammation: common themes and therapeutic opportunities. *Seminars in Cancer Biology*, volume 22, 33-40.

40. Michalaki V, et al. (2004). Serum levels of IL-6 and TNF-α correlate with the clinicopatholgoical features and patient survival in patients with prostate cancer. *British Journal of Cancer*, volume 91, 1227.

41. Chung H, et al. (2001). The inflammation hypothesis of aging: molecular modulation by caloric restriction. *Annals of the New York Academy of Science*, volume 928, 327-335.

42. Schroder K, Tschopp, J. (2010). The inflammasomes. *Cell*, volume 140, 821-832.

43. Krabbe K, et al. (2004). Inflammatory mediators in the elderly. *Experimental Gerontology*, volume 39, 687-699.

44. Ferrucci L, et al. (2005). The origins of age-related proinflammatory state. *Blood*, volume 105, 2294-2299.

45. Trayhurn P. (2007). Adipocyte biology. *Obesity Reviews*, volume 8, 41-44.

46. Ortega Martinez de Victoria E. (2009). Macrophage content in subcutaneous adipose tissue: associates with adiposity, age, inflammatory markers, and whole-body insulin action in healthy Pima Indians. *Diabetes*, volume 58, 385-393.

47. Ershler W, Keller E. (2000). Age-associated increased interleukin-6 gene expression, late life diseases, and frailty. *Annual Review of Medicine*, volume 51, 245-270.

48. Straub R. (2007). The complex role of estrogens in inflammation. *Endocrine Reviews*, volume 28(5), 521-574.

49. Maggio M, et al. (2005). The relationship between testosterone and molecular markers of inflammation in older men. *Journal of Endocrinological Investigation*, volume 28, 116-119.

50. Gameiro C, Romao F. (2010). Changes in the immune system during menopause and aging. *Frontiers in Bioscience*, volume 2, 1299-1303.

Chapter 4: Obesity, Microinflammation, and Oxidative Stress

1. Centers for Disease Control and Prevention. *Defining overweight and Obesity*. (2012). Retrieved June 23, 2012, from http://www.cdc.gov/obesity/adult/defining.html.

2. Flegal K, et al. (2010). Prevalence and trends in obesity among US adults. 1999-2008. *Journal of the American Medical Association*, volume 303, 235-241.

3. World Health Organization. *Obesity and overweight*. (2012). Retrieved June 23, 2012, from http://www.who.int/mediacentre/factsheets/fs311/en/.

4. Fox C, et al. (2006). Trends in the incidence of type 2 diabetes mellitus from the 1970s to the 1990s: the Framingham Heart Study. *Circulation*, volume 113, 2914-2918.

5. Stamler R, et al. (1978). Weight and blood pressure: findings in hypertension screening of 1 million Americans. *Journal of the American Medical Association*, volume 240, 1607-1610.

6. Friedman G, et al. (1988). Precursors of essential hypertension: body weight, alcohol and salt use, and parental history of hypertension. *Preventive Medicine*, volume 17, 387-402.

7. Dyer A, et al. (1989). The INTERSALT study: relations of body mass index to blood pressure. *Journal of Human Hypertension*, volume 3, 299-308.

8. Huang Z, et al. (1998). Body weight, weight change, and risk for hypertension in women. *Annals of Internal Medicine*, volume 128, 81-88.

9. Centers for Disease Control and Prevention. *Causes and consequences: what causes overweight and obesity*. (2012). Retrieved June 11, 2012, from http://www.cdc.gov/obesity/adult/causes/index.html.

10. Hotamisligil G, et al. (1995). Increased adipose tissue expression of tumor necrosis factor-α in human obesity and insulin resistance. *Journal of Clinical Investigation*, volume 95, 2409-2415.

11. Berg A, Scherer P. (2005) Adipose tissue, inflammation and cardiovascular disease. *Circulation Research*, volume 96, 939-949.

12. Shoelson S, et al. (2006). Inflammation and insulin resistance. *Journal of Clinical Investigation*, volume 116, 1793-1801.

13. Vozarova B, et al. (2001). Circulating interleukin-6 in relation to adiposity, insulin action and insulin secretion. *Obesity Research*, volume 9, 414-417.

14. Arya S, et al. (2006). C-reactive protein and dietary nutrients in urban Asian Indian adolescents and young adults. *Nutrition*, volume 22, 865-871.

15. Clarke R, et al. (2009). Plasma phospholipid fatty acids and CHD in older men: Whitehall study of London civil servants. *British Journal of Nutrition*, volume 102, 279-284.

16. Mozaffarian D, et al. (2004). Dietary intake of trans-fatty acids and systemic inflammation in women. *American Journal of Clinical Nutrition*, volume 79, 606-612.

17. Lennie T, et al. (2005). Dietary fat intake and proinflammatory cytokine levels in patients with heart failure. *Journal of Cardiac Failure*, volume 11, 613-618.

18. Mozaffarian D, et al. (2009). Health effects fo trans-fatty acids: experimental and observational evidence. *European Journal of Clinical Nutrition*, volume 63, S5-S21.

19. Nettleton J, et al. (2006). Dietary patterns are associated with biochemical markers of inflammation and endothelial activation in the Multi-Ethnic Study of Atherosclerosis (MESA). *American Journal of Clinical Nutrition*, volume 83, 1369-1379.

20. Saghizadeh M, et al. (1996). The expression of TNF- α by human muscle. Relationship to insulin resistance. *Journal of Clinical Investigation*, volume 97, 1111-1116.

21. Cai D, et al. (2005). Local and systemic insulin resistance resulting from hepatic activation of IKK-β and NF- αβ. *Nature Medicine*, volume 11, 183-190.

22. De Souza C, et al. (2005). Consumption of a fat-rich diet activates a proinflammatory response and induces insulin resistance in the hypothalamus. *Eindocrinology*, volume 146, 4192-4199.

23. Ehses J, et al. (2007). Increased number of islet-associated macrophages in type 2 diabetes. *Diabetes*, volume 56, 2356-2370.

24. Weisberg S, et al. (2003). Obesity is associated with macrophage accumulation in adipose tissue. *Journal of Clinical Investigation*, volume 112, 1796-1808.

25. Xu H, et al. (2003). Chronic inflammation in fat plays a crucial role in the development of obesity-related insulin resistance. *Journal of Clinical Investigation*, volume 112, 1821-1830.

26. Liu J, et al. (2009). Genetic deficiency and pharmacological stabilization of mast cells reduce diet-induced obesity and diabetes in mice. *Nature Medicine*, volume 15, 940-945.

27. Ohmura K, et al. (2010). Natural killer T cells are involved in adipose tissues inflammation and glucose intolerance in diet-induced obese mice. *Arteriosclerosis Thrombosis Vascular Biology*, volume 30, 193-199.

28. Mohanty P, et al. (2002). Both lipid and protein intakes stimulate generation of reactive oxygen species by polymorphonuclear leukocytes

and mononuclear cells. *American Journal of Clinical Nutrition*, volume 75, 767-772.

29. Singh R, et al. (1998). Association of low plasma concentrations of antioxidant vitamins, magnesium and zinc with high body fat per cent measured by bioelectrical impedance analysis in Indian men. *Magnesium Research*, volume 11, 3-10.

30. Decsi T, et al. (1997). Reduced plasma concentrations of alpha-tocopherol and beta-carotene in obese boys. *Journal of Pediatrics*, volume 130, 653-655.

31. Ohrvall M, et al. (1993). Lower tocopherol serum levels in subjects with abdominal adiposity. *Journal of Internal Medicine*, volume 234, 53-60.

32. Dandona P, et al. (2001). The suppressive effect of dietary restriction and weight loss in the obese on the generation of reactive oxygen species by leukocytes, lipid peroxidation, and protein carbonylation. *Journal of Clinical Endocrinology and Metabolism*, volume 86, 355-362.

33. Dandona P, et al. (2001). Inhibitory effect of a two-day fast on reactive oxygen species (ROS) generation by leucocytes and plasma ortho-tyrosine and meta-tyrosine concentrations. *Journal of Clinical Endocrinology and Metabolism*, volume 86, 2899-2902.

34. Hotamisligil G, et al. (1994). Tumor necrosis factor α inhibits signaling from the insulin receptor. *Proceedings of the National Academy of Sciences USA*, volume 91, 4854-4858.

35. Stephens J, et al. (1997). Tumor necrosis factor α-induced insulin resistance in 3T3-L1 adipocytes is accompanied by a loss of insulin receptor substrate-1 and GLUT4 expression without a loss of insulin receptor-

mediated signal transduction. *Journal of Biological Chemistry*, volume 272, 971-976.

36. Engelman J, et al. (2000). Tumor necrosis factor α-mediated insulin resistance, but not dedifferentiation is abrogated by MEK1/2 inhibitors in 3T3-L1 adipocytes. *Molecular Endocrinology*, volume 14, 1557-1569.

37. Boura-Halfon S, Zick Y. (2009). Phosphorylation of IRS preteins, insulin action, and insulin resistance. *American Journal of Physiology-Endocrinology and Metabolism*, volume 296, E581-591.

38. Kopp H, et al (2003). Impact of weight loss on inflammatory proteins and their association with the insulin resistance syndrome in morbidly obese patients. *Arteriosclerosis Thrombosis and Vascular Biology*, volume 23, 1042-1047.

39. McLaughlin T, et al. (2002). Differentiation between obesity and insulin resistance in the association with C-reactive protein. *Circulation*, volume 106, 2908-2912.

40. Vazquez L, et al. (2005). Effects of changes in body weight and insulin resistance on inflammation and endothelial function in morbid obesity after bariatric surgery. *Journal of Clinical Endocrinology and Metabolism*, volume 90, 316-322.

41. Kopp H, et al. (2005). Effects of marked weight loss on plasma levels of adiponectin, markers of chronic subclinical inflammation and insulin resistance in morbidly obese women. *International Journal of Obesity*, volume 29, 766-771.

42. Cai D, et al. (2005). Local and systemic insulin resistance resulting from hepatic activation of IKK-β and NF-κB. *Nature Medicine*, volume 11, 183-190.

43. Baffy G. (2009). Kupffer cells in non-alcoholic fatty liver disease: the emerging view. *Journal of Hepatology*, volume 51, 212-223.

44. Feinstein R, et al. (1993). Tumor necrosis factor α suppresses insulin-induced tyrosine phosphorylation of insulin receptor and its substrates. *Journal of Biological Chemistry*, volume 268, 26055-26058.

45. Feingold K, et al. (1987). Tumor necrosis factor-α stimulates hepatic lipogenesis in the rat in vivo. *Journal of Clinical Investigation*, volume 80, 184-190.

46. Ehses J, et al. (2007). Increased number of islet-associated macrophages in type 2 diabetes. *Diabetes*, volume 56, 2356-2370.

47. Giannoukakis N, et al (2000). Protection of human islets from the effects of interleukin-1β by adenoviral gene transfer of an IκB repressor. *Journal of Biological Chemistry*, volume 275, 36509-36513.

48. Christiansen T, et al. (2005). Monocyte chemoattractant protein-1 is produced in isolated adipocytes, associated with adiposity and reduced after weight loss in morbid obese subjects. *International Journal of Obesity and Related Metabolic Disorders*, volume 29, 146-150.

49. Kamei N, et al. (2006). Overexpression of monocyte chemoattractant protein-1 in adipose tissues causes macrophage recruitment and insulin resistance. *Journal of Biological Chemistry*, volume 281, 26602-26614.

50. Bergstrom A, et al. (2001). Overweight as an avoidable cause of cancer in Europe. *International Journal of Cancer*, volume 91, 421-430.

51. World Cancer Research Fund (2007). *Food, nutrition, physical activity, and the prevention of cancer: a global perspective.* Washington: American Institute for Cancer Research.

52. MacInnis R, English D. (2006). Body size and composition and prostate cancer risk: systematic review and met-regression analysis. *Cancer Causes and Control*, volume 17, 989-1003.

53. Carmichael A. (2006). Obesity and prognosis of breast cancer. *Obesity Reviews*, volume 7(4), 333-340.

54. Dignam J, et al. (2006). Body mass index and outcome sin patients who receive adjuvant chemotherapy for colon cancer. *Journal of the National Cancer Institute*, volume 98, 1647-1654.

55. Kjaerbye-Thygesen A, et al. (2006). Smoking and overweight: negative prognostic factors in stage III epithelial ovarian cancer. *Cancer Epidemiology Biomarkers and Prevention*, volume 15, 798-803.

56. von Gruenigen V, et al. (2006). Treatment effects, disease recurrence, and survival in obese women with early endometrial carcinoma: a Gynecologic Oncology Group study. *Cancer*, volume 107, 2786-2791.

57. Bruning P, et al. (1992). Insulin resistance and breast cancer risk. *International Journal of Cancer*, volume 52, 511-516.

58. Hirose K, et al. (2003). Insulin, insulin-like growth factor-1 and breast cancer risk in Japanese women. *Asian Pacific Journal of Cancer Prevention*, volume 4, 239-246.

59. Lukanova A, et al. (2004). Prediagnostic levels of C-peptide, IGF-I, IGFBP-1, -2, -3 and risk of endometrial cancer. *International Journal of Cancer*, volume 108, 262-268.

60. Wei E, et al. (2005). A prospective study of C-peptide, insulin-like growth factor-I, insuin-like growth factor binding protein-1 and the risk of colorectal cancer in women. *Cancer Epidemiological Biomarkers Preview*, volume 14, 850-855.

61. Lindblad P, et al. (1999). The role of diabetes mellitus in the aetiology of renal cell cancer. *Diabetologia*, volume 42, 107-117.

62. Larsson S, et al. (2005). Diabetes mellitus and risk of colorectal cancer: a meta-analysis. *International Journal of Cancer*, volume 97, 1679-1687.

63. Huxley R, et al. (2005). Type-II diabetes and pancreatic cancer: a meta-analysis of 36 studies. *British Journal of Cancer*, volume 92, 2076-2083.

64. Friberg E, et al. (2007). Diabetes mellitus and risk of endometrial cancer: a meta-analysis. *Diabetologia*, volume 50, 1365-1374.

65. Renehan A, et al. (2006). Obesity and cancer risk: the role of insulin-IGF axis. *Trends in Endocrinology and Metabolism*, volume 17, 328-336.

66. Chan J, et al. (1998). Plasm insulin-like growth factor-1 and prostate cancer risk: a prospective study. *Science*, volume 279, 563-566.

67. Hankinson S, et al. (1998). Circulating conenctraqtions of insulin-like growth factor-1 and risk of breast cancer. *Lancet*, volume 351, 1393-1396.

68. Ma J, et al. (1999). Prospective study of colorectal cancer risk in men andplasma levels of insuin-like growth factor-I (IGF-I) and IGF-binding protein-3. *Journal of the National Cancer Institute*, volume 91, 620-625.

69. Samani, A. et al. (2007). The role of the IGF system in cancer growth and metastasis: overview and recent insights. *Endocrine Reviews*, volume 28, 20-47.

70. Hong O, et al. (2007). Hyperglycemia and hyperinsulinemia have additive effects on activation and proliferation of pancreatic stellate cells:

possible explanation of islet-specific fibrosis in type 2 diabetes mellitus. *Journal of Cell Biochemistry*, volume 101, 665-675.

71. Renehan A, et al. (2008). Obesity and cancer: Pathophysiological and biological mechanisms. *Archives of Physiology and Biochemistry*, volume 114, 71-83.

72. Kelesidis T, et al. (2010). Narrative review: the role of leptin in human physiology: emerging clinical applications. *Annals of Internal Medicine*, volume 152, 93-100.

73. Garofalo C, Surmacz, E. (2006). Leptin and cancer. *Journal of Cell Physiology*, volume 207, 12-22.

74. Trayhurn P, Wood I. (2004). Adipokines: inflammation and the pleiotropic role of white adipose tissue. *British Journal of Nutrition*, volume 92, 347-355.

75. Sierra-Honigmann M, et al. (1998). Biological action of leptin as an angiogenic factor. *Science*, volume 281, 1683-1686.

76. Urbancsek J, et al. (2002). Impact of obesity and leptin levels on the secretion of estradiol, inhibin A and B, during ovarian stimulation with gonadotropins. *Gynecological Endocrinology*, volume 16, 285-292.

77. Maccio A, et al. (2010). Correlation of body mass index and leptin with tumor size and stage of disease in hormone-dependent postmenopausal breast cancer: preliminary results and therapeutic implications. *Journal of Molecular Medicine*, volume 88, 677-686.

78. Rose D, et al. (2004). Obesity, adipocytokines, and insulin resistance in breast cancer. *Obesity Reviews*, volume 5, 153-165.

79. Stattin P, et al. (2003). Plasma leptin and colorectal cancer risk: a prospective study in Northern Sweden. *Oncology Reports*, volume 10(6), 2015-2021.

80. Stattin P, et al. (2004). Obesity and colon cancer: does leptin provide a link? *International Journal of Cancer*, volume 109, 149-152.

81. Tamakoshi K, et al. (2005). Leptin is associated with an increased female colorectal cancer risk: a nested case-control study in Japan. *Oncology*, volume 68, 454-461.

82. Engeland A, et al. (2006). Body size and thyroid cancer in two million Norwegian men and women. *British Journal of Cancer*, volume 95, 366-370.

83. Akinci M, et al. (2009). Leptin levels in thyroid cancer. *Asian Journal of Surgery*, volume 32, 216-223.

84. Clavel-Chapelon F, et al. (2010). Risk of differentiated thyroid cancer in relation to adult weight, height and body shape for life: the French E3N cohort. *International Journal of Cancer*, volume 126, 2984-2990.

85. Leitzmann M, et al. Prospective study of body mass index, physical activity and thyroid cancer. *International Journal of Cancer*, volume 126, 2947-2956.

86. Fasshauer M, et al. (2002). Hormonal regulation of adiponectin gene expression in 3T3-L1 adipocytes. *Biochemical and Biophysical Research Communications*, volume 290, 1084-1089.

87. Ahima R, (2006). Adipose tissue as an endocrine organ. *Obesity*, volume 14, 242S-249S.

88. Brakenhielm E, et al. (2004). Adipoenectin-induced antiangiogenesis and antitumor activity involve caspase-mediated endothelial cell apoptosis. *Proceedings of the National Academy of Sciences USA*, volume 101, 2476-2481.

89. Miyoshi Y, et al. (2003). Association of serum adiponectin levels with breast cancer risk. *Clinical Cancer Research*, volume 9, 5699-5704.

90. Mantzoros C, et al. (2004). Adiponectin and breast cancer risk. *Journal of Clinical Endocrinology and Metabolism*, volume 89, 1102-1107.

91. Petridou E, et al. (2003). Plasma adiponectin concentrations in relation to endometrial cancer: a case-control study in Greece. *Journal of Clinical Endocrinology and Metabolism*, volume 88, 993-997.

92. Dal Maso L, et al. (2004). Circulating adiponectin and endometrial cancer risk. *Journal of Clinical Endocrinology and Metabolism,* volume 89, 1160-1163.

93. Soliman P, et al. (2006). Association between adiponectin, insulin resistance, and endometrial cancer. *Cancer*, volume 106, 2376-2381.

94. Cust A, et al. (2007). Plasma adiponectin levels and endometrial cancer risk in pre- and postmenopausal women. *Journal of Clinical Endocrinology and Metabolism*, volume 92, 255-263.

95. Otake S, et al. (2005). Association of visceral fat accumulation and plasma adiponectin with colorectal adenoma: evidence for participation of insulin resistance. *Clinical Cancer Research*, volume 11, 3642-3646.

96. Wei E, et al. (2005). Low plasma adiponectin levels and risk of colorectal cancer in a men: a prospective study. *Journal of the National Cancer Institute*, volume 97, 1688-1694.

97. Yamaji T, et al. (2010). Interaction between adiponectin and leptin influences the risk of colorectal adenoma. *Cancer Research*, volume 70, 5430-5437.

98. Goktas S, et al. (2005). Prostate cancer and adiponectin. *Urology*, volume 65, 1168-1172.

99. Ishikawa M, et al. (2005). Plasma adiponectin and gastric cancer. *Clinical Cancer Research*, volume 11, 466-472.

100. Renehan A. (2008). *Hormones, Growth Factors and Tumor Growth*. Hay I, Wass J, editors. Oxford: Oxford University.

101. Key T, et al. (2003). Body mass index, serum sex hormones and breast cancer risk in postmenopausal women. *Journal of the National Cancer Institute*, volume 95, 1218-1226.

102. Kaaks R, et al. (2005). Postmenopausal serum androgens, oestrogens and breast cancer risk: the European prospective investigation into cancer and nutrition. *Endocrine-Related Cancer*, volume 12, 1071-1082.

103. Thune I, et al. (1997). Physical activity and the risk of breast cancer. *New England Journal of Medicine*, volume 336, 1269-1275.

104. Eliassen A, et al. (2010). Physical activity and risk of breast cancer among postmenopausal women. *Archives of Internal Medicine*, volume 170, 1758-1764.

105. Campbell K, et al. (2012). Reduced-calorie dietary weight loss, exercise, and sex hormones in postmenopausal women: randomized controlled trial. *Journal of Clinical Oncology*, volume 30, 2314-2326.

106. Calle E, Kaaks R. (2004). Overweight, obesity and cancer: epidemiological evidence and proposed mechanisms. *Nature Reviews Cancer*, volume 4, 579-591.

107. d'Addadi Fagagna F, et al. (2003). A DNA damage checkpoint response in telomere-initiated senescence. *Nature*, volume 426, 194-198.

108. Blasco M. (2005). Telomeres and human disease: ageing, cancer and beyond. *Nature Reviews Genetics*, volume 6, 611-622.

109. von Zglinicki T. (2002). Oxidative stress shortens telomeres. *Trends in Biochemical Sciences*, volume 27, 339-344.

110. Demissie S, et al. (2006). Insulin resistance, oxidative stress, hypertension, and leukocyte telomere length in men from the Framingham Heart Study. *Aging Cell*, volume 5, 325-330.

111. Matthews C, et al. (2006). Vascular smooth muscle cells undergo telomere-based senescence in human atherosclerosis: effects of telomerase and oxidative stress. *Circulation Research*, volume 99, 156-164.

112. Haendeler J, et al. (2004). Antioxidants inhibit nuclear export of telomerase reverse transcriptase and delay replicative senescence of endothelial cells. *Circulation Research*, volume 94, 768-775.

113. Aviv A, et al. (2006). Menopause modifies the association of leukocyte telomere length with insulin resistance and inflammation. *Journal of Clinical Endocrinology and Metabolism*, volume 91, 635-640.

114. Carrerro J, et al. (2008). Telomere attrition is associated with inflammation, low fetuin-A levels and high mortality in prevalent haemodialysis patients. *Journal of Internal Medicine*, volume 263, 302-312.

115. Valdes A, et al. (2005). Obesity, cigarette smoking, and telomere length in women. *Lancet*, volume 368, 20-26.

116. Tzanetakou I, et al. (2012). Is obesity linked to aging? Adipose tissue and the role of telomeres. *Ageing Research Reviews*, volume 11, 220-229.

117. Barton M. (2010). Obesity and aging: determinants of endothelial cell dysfunction and atherosclerosis. *Pflügers Archiv European Journal of Physiology*, volume 460, 825-837.

118. Barton M. (2005). Ageing as a determinant of renal and vascular disease: role of endothelial factors. *Nephrology Dialysis Transplantation*, volume 20, 485-490.

119. McCann S, et al. (2005). The nitric oxide theory of aging revisited. *Annals of the New York Academy of Sciences*, volume 1057, 64-84.

Chapter 5: Diabetes, Microinflammation, and Oxidative Stress

1. "Diabetes Basics." *Diabetes Statistics*. American Diabetes Association, 2012. Web. 09 Sept. 2012. <http://www.diabetes.org/diabetes-basics/diabetes-statistics/?loc=DropDownDB-stats>.

2. Treszl A, et al. (2004). Elevated C-reactive protein levels do not correspond to autoimmunity in type 1 diabetes. *Diabetes Care*, volume 27, 2769-2770.

3. Devaraj S, et al. (2007). Evidence of increased inflammation and microcirculatory abnormalities in patients with type 1 diabetes and their role in microvascular complications. *Diabetes*, volume 56, 2790-2796.

4. Pradhan A, et al. (2001). C-reactive protein, interleukin 6 and risk of developing type 2 diabetes mellitus. *Journal of the American Medical Association*, volume 286, 327-334.

5. Voxarova B, et al. (2002). High white blood cell count is associated with a worsening of insulin sensitivity and predicts the development of type 2 diabetes. *Diabetes*, volume 51, 455-461.

6. Thorand B, et al. (2003). C-reactive protein as a predictor for incident diabetes mellitus among middle-aged men: Results from the MON-ICA Augsburg cohort study, 1984-1998. *Archives of Internal Medicine*, volume 163, 93-99.

7. Hotamisligil G, et al. (1993). Adipose expression of tumor-necrosis-factor-alpha—direct role in obesity-linked insulin resistance. *Science*, volume 259, 87-91.

8. Goldberg R. (2009). Cytokine and cytokine-like inflammation markers, endothelial dysfunction, and imbalanced coagulation in development of diabetes and its complications. *Journal of Clinical Endocrinology and Metabolism*, volume 94, 3171-3182.

9. Duncan B, et al. (1999). Factor VIII and other hemostasis variables are related to incident diabetes in adults. The Atherosclerosis Risk in Communities (ARIC) Study. *Diabetes Care*, volume 22, 767-772.

10. Schmidt M, et al. (1999). Markers of inflammation and prediction of diabetes mellitus in adults (Atherosclerosis Risk in Communities study): a cohort study. *Lancet*, volume 353, 1649-1652.

11. Festa A. et al. (2002). Elevated levels of acute-phase proteins and plasminogen activator inhibitor-1 predict the development of type 2 diabetes: the insulin resistance atherosclerosis study. *Diabetes*, volume 51, 1131-1137.

12. Liu S, et al. (2007). A prospective study of inflammatory cytokines and diabetes mellitus in a multiethnic cohort of postmenopausal women. *Archives of Internal Medicine*, volume 167, 1676-1685.

13. Lindsay R, et al. (2002). Adiponectin and development of type 2 diabetes in the Pima Indian population. *Lancet*, volume 360, 57-58.

14. Duncan B, et al. (2004). Adiponectin and the development of type 2 diabetes. The Atherosclerosis Risk in Communities Study. *Diabetes*, volume 53, 2473-2478.

15. Daimon M, et al. (2003). Decreased serum levels of adiponectin are a risk factor for the progression to type 2 diabetes in the Japanese population: the Funagata study. *Diabetes Care*, volume 26, 2015-2020.

16. Spranger J, et al. (2003). Adiponectin and protection against type 2 diabetes mellitus. *Lancet*, volume 361, 226-228.

17. Snehalatha C, et al. (2003). Plasma adiponectin is an independent predictor of type 2 diabetes in Asian Indians. *Diabetes Care*, volume 26, 3226-3229.

18. Ghiselli A, et al. (1992). Salicylate hydroxylation as an early marker of in vivo oxidative stress in diabetic patients. *Free Radical Biology and Medicine*, volume 13, 621-626.

19. Gopaul N, et al. (1995). Plasma 8-epi-PGF2 alpha levels are levated in indviduals with non-insulin dependent diabetes mellitus. *Federation of European Biochemical Societies Letters*, volume 368, 225-229.

20. Shin C, et al. (2001). Serum 8-hydroxy-quanine levels are increased in diabetic patients. *Diabetes Care*, volume 24, 733-737.

21. Murakami K, et al. (1989). Impairment of glutathione metabolism in erythrocytes from patients with diabetes mellitus. *Metabolism*, volume 38, 753-758.

22. Sharma A, et al. (2000). Evaluation of oxidative stress before and after control of glycemia and after vitamin E supplementation in diabetic patients. *Metabolism*, volume 49, 160-162.

23. Sakuraba H, et al. (2002). Reduced beta-cell mass and expression of oxidative stress-related DNA damage in the islet of Japanese type II diabetic patients. *Diabetologia*, volume45, 85-96.

24. Harris M, et al. (1992). Onset of NIDDM occurs at least 4-7 yr before clinical diagnosis. *Diabetes Care*, volume 15, 815-819.

25. Pisani P, (2008). Hyperinsulinemia and cancer, meta-analyses of epidemiological studies. *Archives of Physiology and Biochemistry*, volume 114, 63-70.

26. Pollak M. (2008). Insulin and insulin-like growth factor signaling in neoplasia. *Nature Reviews Cancer*, volume 8, 915-928.

27. Frasca F, et al. (1999). Insulin receptor isoform A, a newly recognized, high affinity insulin-like growth factor II receptor in fetal and cancer cells. *Molecular Cell Biology*, volume 19, 3278-3288.

28. Vella V, et al. (2002). A novel autocrine loop involving IGF-II and the insulin receptor isoform-A stimulates growth of thyroid cancer. *Journal of Clinical Endocrinology and Metabolism*, volume 87, 245-254.

29. Laporte D, et al. (2011). Metabolic status rather than cell cycle signals control quiescence entry and exit. *Journal of Cell Biology*, volume 192, 949-957.

30. Tannock I, et al. (1986). Influence of glucose concentration on growth and formation of necrosis in spheroids derived from a human bladder cancer cell line. *Cancer Research*, volume 46, 3105-3110.

31. Warburg O. (1956). On the origin of cancer cells. *Science*, volume 123, 309-314.

32. Muti P, et al. (2002). Fasting glucose is a risk factor for breast cancer: a prospective study. *Cancer Epidemiology, Biomarkers & Prevention*, volume 11, 1361-1368.

33. Jee S, et al. (2005). Fasting serum glucose level and cancer risk in Korean men and women. *Journal of the American Medical Association*, volume 293, 194-2002.

34. Stattin P, et al. (2007). Prospective study of hyperglycemia and cancer risk. *Diabetes Care*, volume 30, 561-567.

35. Stocks T, et al. (2009). Blood glucose and risk of incident and fatal cancer in the metabolic syndrome and cancer project (mecan): analysis of six prospective cohorts. *PLOS Medicine*, volume 6: e1000201.

36. Liao S, et al. (2010). Type 2 diabetes mellitus and characteristics of breast cancer in China. *Asian Pacific Journal of Cancer Prevention*, volume 11, 933-937.

37. Larsson S, et al. (2007). Diabetes mellitus and risk of breast cancer: a meta-analysis. *International Journal of Cancer*, volume 121, 856-862.

38. Michels K, et al. (2003). Type 2 diabetes and subsequent incidence of breast cancer in the Nurses' Health Study. *Diabetes Care*, volume 26, 1752-1758.

39. Wolf I, et al. (2005). Diabetes mellitus and breast cancer. *Lancet Oncology*, volume 6, 103-111.

40. Srowkowski T, et al. (2009). Impact of diabetes mellitus on complications and outcomes of adjuvant chemotherapy in older patients with breast cancer. *Journal of Clinical Oncology*, volume 27, 2170-2176.

41. "Pancreatic Cancer." *US News*. U.S.News & World Report, Sept.-Oct. 2009. Web. 17 Sept. 2012. <http://health.usnews.com/health-conditions/cancer/pancreatic-cancer>.

42. Baghurst P, et al. (1991). A case-control study of diet and cancer of the pancreas. *American Journal of Epidemiology*, volume 134, 167-179.

43. Berrington de Gonzalez A, et al. (2003). A meta-analysis of obesity and the risk of pancreatic cancer. *British Journal of Cancer*, volume 89, 519-523.

44. Everhart J, Wright D. (1995). Diabetes mellitus as a risk factor for pancreatic cancer: a meta-analysis. *Journal of the American Medical Association*, volume 273, 1605-1609.

45. Huxley R, et al. (2005). Type-II diabetes and pancreatic cancer: a meta-analysis of 36 studies. *British Journal of Cancer*, volume 92, 2076-2083.

46. Want F, et al. (2006). Diabetes mellitus and pancreatic cancer in a population-based case-control study in the San Francisco Bay Area, California. *Cancer Epidemiology, Biomarkers & Prevention*, volume 15, 1458-1463.

47. Limburg P, et al. (2006). Clinically confirmed type 2 diabetes mellitus and colorectal cancer risk: a population-based retrospective cohort study. *American Journal of Gastroenterology*, volume 101, 1872-1879.

48. Deng L, et al. (2012). Diabetes mellitus and the incidence of colorectal cancer: an updated systematic review and meta-analysis. *Digestive Diseases and Sciences*, volume 57, 1576-1585.

49. Yang Y, et al. (2004). Insulin therapy and colorectal cancer risk among type 2 diabetes mellitus patients. *Gastroenterology*, volume 127, 1044-1050.

50. Nagel J, Goke B. (2006). [Colorectal carcinoma screening in patients with type 2 diabetes mellitus]. *Zeitschrift für Gastroenterologie*, volume 44, 1153-1165.

51. Chung Y, et al. (2008). Insulin therapy and colorectal adenoma risk among patients with type 2 diabetes mellitus: a case-control study in Korea. *Diseases of the Colon and Rectum*, volume 51, 593-597.

52. El-Serag H, et al. (2006). The association between diabetes and hepatocellular carcinoma: a systematic review of epidemiologic evidence. *Clinical Gastroenterology and Hepatology*, volume 4, 369-380.

53. Lai M, et al. (2006). Type 2 diabetes and hepatocellular carcinoma: a cohort study in high prevalence area of hepatitis virus infection. *Hepatology*, volume 43, 1295-1302.

54. Wang P, et al. (2012). Diabetes mellitus and risk of hepatocellular carcinoma: a systematic review and meta-analysis. *Diabetes/Metabolism Research and Reviews*, volume 28, 109.

55. Anderson K, et al. (2001). Diabetes and endometrial cancer in the Iowa women's health study. *Cancer Epidemiology, Biomarkers & Prevention*, volume 10, 611-616.

56. Friberg E, et al. (2007). Diabetes mellitus and risk of endometrial cancer: a meta-analysis. *Diabetologia*, volume 50, 1365-1374.

57. Lindblad P, et al. (1999). The role of diabetes mellitus in the etiology of renal cell cancer. *Diabetologia*, volume 42, 107-112.

58. Larsson S, Wolk, A. (2011). Diabetes mellitus and incidence of kidney cancer: a meta-analysis of cohort studies. *Diabetologia*, volume 54, 1013-1018.

59. Mitri J, et al. (2008). Diabetes and risk of non-Hodgkin's lymphoma. *Diabetes Care*, volume 31, 2391-2397.

60. DeCensi A, et al. (2010). Metformin and cancer risk in diabetic patients: a systematic review and meta-analysis. *Cancer Prevention Research*, volume 3, 1451-1461.

61. Noto H, et al. (2012). Cancer risk in diabetic patients treated with metformin: a systematic review and meta-analysis. *PLOS ONE*, volume 7: e33411. Doi: 10.1371/journal.pone.0033411.

62. "Cardiovascular Disease & Diabetes." *Cardiovascular Disease & Diabetes*. N.p., n.d. Web. 21 Sept. 2012. <http://www.heart.org/HEARTORG/Conditions/Diabetes/WhyDiabetesMatters/Cardiovascular-Disease-Diabetes_UCM_313865_Article.jsp>.

63. Brownlee M. (1995). Advanced glycosylation in diabetes and gain. *Annual Review of Medicine*, volume 46, 223-234.

64. Reddy S, et al. (1996). Carboxymethyllysine is a dominant AGE antigen in tissue proteins. *Biochemistry*, volume 34, 10872-10878.

65. Palinski W, et al. (1995). Immunological presence of AGEs in atherosclerotic lesions of euglycemic rabbits. *Arteriosclerosis, Thrombosis, and Vascular Biology*, volume 15, 571-582.

66. Horie K, et al. (1997). Immunohistochemical colocalization of glycoxidation products and lipid peroxidation products in diabetic renal glomerular lesions. *Journal of Clinical Investigation*, volume 100, 2995-3004.

67. Schmidt A, et al. (1994). Cellular receptors for AGEs. *Arteriosclerosis and Thrombosis*, volume 14, 1521-1528.

68. Semenkovich C, Heinecke J. (1997). The mystery of diabetes and atherosclerosis. *Diabetes*, volume 46, 327-334.

69. Neeper M, et al. (1999). Cloning and expression of RAGE: a cell surface receptor for advanced glycosylation end products of proteins. *Journal of Biological Chemistry*, volume 267, 14998-15004.

70. Schmidt A, et al. (2001). The multiligand receptor RAGE as a progression factor amplifying immune and inflammatory response. *Journal of Clinical Investigation*, volume 108, 949-955.

71. Schmidt A, Stern D. (2000). RAGE: a new target for the prevention and treatment of the vascular and inflammatory complications of diabetes. *Trends in Endocrinology and Metabolism*, volume 11, 368-375.

72. Haitoglou C, et al. (1992). Altered cellular interactions between endothelial cells and nonenzymatically glucosylated laminin/type IV collagen. *Journal of Biological Chemistry*, volume 267, 12404-12407.

73. Brownlee M. (1995). Advanced protein glycosylation in diabetes and aging. *Annual Review of Medicine*, volume 46, 223-234.

74. Bucala R. (1994). Modification of low-density lipoprotein by advanced glycation end products contributes to the dyslipidemia of diabetes and renal insufficiency. *Proceedings of the National Academy of Sciences USA*, volume 91, 9441-9445.

75. Gempel K, et al. (1993). In-vitro carboxymethylation of low-density lipoptorein alters its metabolism via the high-affinity receptor. *Hormone and Metabolic Research*, volume 25, 250-252.

76. Bucala R, et al. (1991). Advanced glycosylation products quench nitric oxide and mediate defective endothelium-dependent vasodilatation in experimental diabetes. *Journal of Clinical Investigation*, volume 87, 432-438.

77. Schmidt A, et al. (1994). Receptor for advanced glycation end products (AGEs) has a central role in vessel wall interactions and gene activation in response to circulating AGE proteins. *Proceedings of the National Academy of Sciences USA*, volume 91, 8807-8811.

78. Basta G, et al. (2004). Advanced glycation end products and vascular inflammation: implications for accelerated atherosclerosis in diabetes. *Cardiovascular Research*, volume 63, 582-592.

79. Edelstein D, et al. (1992). Mechanistic studies of advanced glycosylation end product inhibition by aminoguanidine. *Diabetes*, volume 41, 26-29.

80. Iwashima Y, et al. (2000). Advanced glycation end products-induced gene expression of scavenger receptors in cultured human monocyte-derived macrophages. *Biochemical and Biophysical Research Communications*, volume 277, 368-380.

81. Franco O, et al. (2007). Associations of diabetes mellitus with total life expectancy and life expectancy with and without cardiovascular disease. *Archives of Internal Medicine*, volume 167, 1145-1151.

82. Pollreisz A, Schmidt-Erfurth S. (2010). Diabetic Cataract—pathogenesis, epidemiology and treatment. *Journal of Ophthalmology*, volume 2010, Article ID 608751, 8 pages, doi: 10.1155/3010/608751.

83. Penson D, Wessels H. (2004). Erectile dysfunction in diabetic patients. *Diabetes Spectrum*, volume 17, 225-230.

84. Kawamura T, et al. (2012). Cognitive impairment in diabetic patients: can diabetic control prevent cognitive decline? *Journal of Diabetes Investigation*, doi: 10.1111/j.2040-1124.2012.00234.x.

85. Giovannucci E, et al. (2010). Diabetes and cancer: a consensus report. *Diabetes Care*, volume 33, 1674-1685.

86. Goldin A, et al. (2006). Advanced glycation end products: sparking the development of diabetic vascular injury. *Circulation*, volume 114, 597-605.

87. Krajcovicova-Kudlackova M, et al. (2002). Advanced glycation end products and nutrition. *Physiological Research*, volume 51, 313-316.

88. Murrillo-Ortiz B, et al. (2012). Telomore length and type 2 diabetes in males, a premature aging syndrome. *Aging Male*, volume 15, 54-58.

89. Monickaraj F, et al. (2012). Accelerated aging as evidenced by increased telomere shortening and mitochondrial DNA depletion in patients with type 2 diabetes. *Molecular and Cellular Biochemistry*, volume 365, 343-350.

Chapter 6: Treating Microinflammation and Oxidative Stress—Primary Prevention of Aging and Disease

1. Mahdi J, et al. (2006). The historical analysis of aspirin discovery, its relation to the willow tree and antiproliferative and anticancer potential. *Cell Proliferation*, volume 39, 147-155.

2. Sandler R, et al. (2003). A randomized trial of aspirin to prevent colorectal adenomas in patients with previous colorectal cancer. *New England Journal of Medicine*, volume 348, 883-890.

3. Benamouzig R, et al. (2003). Daily soluble aspirin and prevention of colorectal adenoma recurrence: one-year results of the APACC Trial. *Gastroenterology*, volume 125, 32-336.

4. Baron J, et al. (2003). A randomized trial of aspirin to prevent colorectal adenomas. *New England Journal of Medicine*, volume 348, 891-899.

5. Logan R, et al. (2008). Aspirin and folic acid for the prevention of recurrent colorectal adenomas. *Gastroenterology*, volume 134, 29-38.

6. Chan A, et al. (2004). A prospective study of aspirin use and the risk for colorectal adenoma. *Annals of Internal Medicine*, volume 140, 157-166.

7. Chan A, et al (2005). Long-term use of aspirin and nonsteroidal anti-inflammatory drugs and risk of colorectal cancer. *Journal of the American Medical Association*, volume 294(8), 914-923.

8. Rothwell P, et al. (2011). Effect of daily aspirin on long-term risk of death due to cancer: analysis of individual patient data from randomised trials. *Lancet*, volume 377, 31-41.

9. Weber C, et al. (1995). Aspirin inhibits nuclear factor-κB mobilization and monocyte adhesion in stimulated human endothelial cells. *Circulation*, volume 91, 1914-1917.

10. Ikonomidis I, et al. (1999). Increased proinflammatory cytokines in patients with chronic stable angina and their reduction by aspirin. *Circulation*, volume 100(8), 793-798.

11. Solheim S, et al. (2003). Influence of aspirin on inflammatory markers in patients after acute myocardial infarction. *American Journal of Cardiology*, volume 92(7), 843-845.

12. Serhan C, et al. (2002). Resolvins: a family of bioactive products of omega-3 fatty acid transformation circuits initiated by aspirin treatment that counter proinflammation signals. *Journal of Experimental Medicine*, volume 196(8), 1025-1037.

13. Arber N, et al. (2006). Celecoxib for the prevention of colorectal adenomatous polyps. *New England Journal of Medicine*, volume 355(9), 885-895.

14. Bertagnolli M, et al. (2006). Celecoxib for the prevention of sporadic colorectal adenomas. *New England Journal of Medicine*, volume 355, 873-884.

15. Baron J, et al. (2006). A randomized trial of rofecoxib for the chemo-prevention of colorectal adenomas. *Gastroenterology*, volume 131, 1674-1682.

16. Solomon S, et al. (2008). Cardiovascular risk of celecoxib in 6 random-ized placebo-controlled trials: the cross trial safety analysis. *Circulation*, volume 117(16), 2104-2113.

17. Giardello F, et al. (1993). Treatment of colonic and rectal adenomas with sulindac in familial adenomatous polyposis. *New England Journal of Medicine*, volume 328(18), 1313-1316.

18. Labayle D, et al. (1991). Sulindac causes regression of rectal polyps in familial adenomatous polyposis. *Gastroenterology*, volume 101(3), 635-539.

19. Meyskens C, et al (2008). Difluoromethylornithine plus sulindac for the prevention of sporadic colorectal adenomas: a randomized placebo-con-trolled, double-blind trial. *Cancer Prevention Research*, volume 1(1), 32-38.

20. Johannesdottir S, et al. (2012). Nonsteroidal anti-inflammatory drugs and the risk of skin cancer: A population-based case-control study. *Can-cer*, May 29. doi: 10.1002/cncr.27406.

21. Hepgul G, et al. (2010). Preventive effect of pentoxifylline on acute radiation damage via antioxidant and anti-inflammatory pathways. *Digestive Disease Science*, volume 55(3), 617-625.

22. Goicoechea M, et al. (2012). Effects of pentoxifylline on inflammatory parameters in chronic kidney disease patients: a randomized trial. *Jour-nal of Nephrology*, epub Jan 11.

23. Gupta S, et al. (2010). Anti-inflammatory treatment with pentoxi-fylline improves HIV-related endothelial dysfunction: a pilot study. *AIDS*, volume 24(9), 1377-80.

24. Maiti R, et al. (2007). Effect of pentoxifylline on inflammatory burden, oxidative stress and platelet aggregability in hypertensive type 2 diabetes mellitus patients. *Vascular Pharmacology*, volume 47(2-3), 118-124.

25. Pruski M, et al. (2009). Pleiotropic action of short-term metformin and fenofibrate treatment combined with lifestyle intervention, in type 2 diabetic patients with mixed dyslipidemia. *Diabetes Care*, volume 32(8), 1421-1424.

26. The Diabetes Prevention Program Research Group (2005). Intensive lifestyle intervention or metformin on inflammation and coagulation in participants with impaired glucose tolerance. *Diabetes*, volume 54, 1566-1572.

27. Gomez-Garcia A, et al. (2007). [Rosuvastain and metformin decreased inflammation and oxidative stress in patients with hypertension and dyslipidemia. *Revista Española de Cardiologia*, volume 60(12), 1242-1249.

28. Bulcao C, et al. (2007). Effects of simvastatin and metformin on inflammation and insulin resistance in individuals with mild metabolic syndrome. *American Journal of Cardiovascular Drugs*, volume 7(3), 219-224.

29. Weber C, et al. (1997) HMG-CoA reductase inhibitors decrease CD11b expression and CD11b-dependent adhesion of monocytes to endothelium and reduce increased adhesiveness of monocytes isolated from patients with hypercholesterolemia. *Journal of the American College of Cardiology*, volume 30, 1212-1217.

30. Bustos C, et al. (1998). HMG-CoA reductase inhibition by atorvastatin reduces neointimal inflammation in a rabbit model of atherosclerosis. *Journal of the American College of Cardiology*, volume 32, 2057-2064.

31. Ferro D, et al. (2000). Simvastatin inhibits the monocytes expression of proinflammatory cytokines in patients with hypercholesterolemia. *Journal of the American College of Cardiology*, volume 36, 427-431.

32. Mason R, et al. Effects of HMG-CoA reducase inhibitors on endothelial function: role of microdomains and oxidative stress. *Circulation*, volume 109(suppl 1), 1134-1141.

33. Albert M, et al. (2001). Effect of statin therapy on C-reactive protein levels. *Journal of the American Medical Association*, volume 286 (1), 64-70.

34. Ridker P, et al. (2008). Rosuvastatin to prevent vascular events in men and women with elevated C-reactive protein. *New England Journal of Medicine*, volume 359, 2195-2207.

35. Pedersen T, et al. (2000). Follow-up study of patients randomized in the Scandinavian simvastatin survival study (4S) of cholesterol lowering. *American Journal of Cardiology*, volume 86, 257-262.

36. Graaf M, et al. (2004). The risk of cancer in users of statins. *Journal of Clinical Oncology*, volume 22, 2388-2394.

37. Papadakis J, et al. (1999). Coronary events with lipid-lowering therapy: the AFCAPS/TexCAPS trial. Air Force/Texas Coronary Atherosclerosis Prevention Study. *Journal of the American Medical Association*, volume 281, 416-419.

38. Graaf M, et al (2004). Effects of statins and famesyltransferase inhibitors on the development and progression of cancer. *Cancer Treatment Review*, volume 30, 609-641.

39. Wong W, et al. (2002). HMG-CoA reductase inhibitors and the malignant cell: the statin family of drugs as triggers of tumor-specific apoptosis. *Leukemia*, volume 16, 508-519.

40. Kaushal V, et al. (2003). Potential anticancer effects of statins: fact or fiction? *Endothelium*, volume 10, 49-58.

41. Moshfegh A, et al. (2009). What we eat in America, NHANES 2005-2006: usual nutrient intakes from food and water compared to 1997 dietary reference intakes for vitamin D, calcium phosphorus and magnesium. US Department of Agriculture, Agricultural Research Service. Available at http://www.ars.usda.gov/ba/bhnrc/fsrg.

42. Kawata S, et al. (2001). Effect of pravastatin on survival in patients with advanced hepatocellular carcinoma. A randomized controlled trial. *British Journal of Cancer*, volume 84, 886-891.

43. Cauley J, et al. (2003). Lipid-loweirng drug use and breast cancer in older women: a prospective study. *Journal of Women's Health*, volume 12, 749-756.

44. Poynter J, et al. (2005). Statins and the risk of colorectal cancer. *New England Journal of Medicine*, volume 352, 2184-2192.

45. "Magnesium." *Health Professional Fact Sheet*. N.p., n.d. Web. 10 Oct. 2012. <http://ods.od.nih.gov/factsheets/Magnesium-HealthProfessional/>.

46. Barbagall M, et al. (2003). Role of magnesium in insulin action, diabetes and cardio-metabolic syndrome X. *Molecular Aspects in Medicine, volume* 24, 39-52.

47. Touyx R. (2003). Role of magnesium in the pathogenesis of hypertension. *Molecular Aspects in Medicine*, volume 24, 107-136.

48. Rude R, et al. (2009). Skeletal and hormonal effects of magnesium deficiency. *Journal of the American College of Nutrition*, volume 28, 131-141.

49. Leone N, et al. (2006). Zinc, copper and magnesium and risks for all-cause cancer, and cardiovascular mortality. *Epidemiology*, volume 17, 308-314.

50. Abbott R, et al. (2003). Dietary magnesium intake and the future risk of coronary artery disease (The Honolulu Heart Program). *American Journal of Cardiology*, volume 92, 665-669.

51. King E, et al. (2007). Dietary magnesium and C-reactive protein levels in children. *Magnesium Research*, volume 20, 32-36.

52. King D, et al. (2005). Dietary magnesium and C-reactive protein levels. *Journal of the American College of Nutrition*, volume 24, 166-171.

53. Chacko S, et al. (2010). Relations of dietary magnesium intake to biomarkers of inflammation and endothelial dysfunction in an ethnically diverse cohort of postmenopausal women. *Diabetes Care*, volume 33, 304-310.

54. Nettleton J, et al. (2006). Dietary patterns are associated with biochemical markers of inflammation and endothelial activation in the Multi-Ethnic Study of Atherosclerosis (MESA). *American Journal of Clinical Nutrition*, volume 83, 1369-1379.

55. Weglicki W, Philips T. (1992). Pathobiology of magnesium deficiency: a cytokine/neurogenic inflammation hypothesis. *American Journal of Physiology*, volume 263, R734-R737.

56. Weglicki W, et al. (1996). Role of free radicals and substance P in magnesium deficiency. *Cardiovascular Research*, volume 31, 677-682.

57. Mazur A, et al. (2007). Magnesium and the inflammatory response: potential physiopathological implications. *Archives of Biochemistry and Biophysics*, volume 458, 48-56.

58. Blache D, et al (2006). Long-term moderate magnesium deficient diet shows relationships between blood pressure, inflammation and oxidant stress defense in aging rats. *Free Radical Biology and Medicine*, volume 41, 277-284.

59. Rayssiguier Y, et al. (1993). Magnesium and aging: 1. Experimental data: importance of oxidative damage. *Magnesium Research*, volume 6, 373-382.

60. Hans C, et al. (2003). Effect of magnesium supplementation on oxidative stress in alloxanic diabetic rats. *Magnesium Research*, volume 16, 13-19.

61. Yang Y, et al. (2006). Magnesium deficiency enhances hydrogen peroxide production and oxidative damage in chick embryo hepatocye in vitro. *Biometals*, volume 19, 71-81.

62. Afanas'ev I, et al. (1995). Study of antioxidant properties of metal aspartates. *Analyst*, volume 120, 859-862.

63. Ma J, et al. (1995). Associations of serum and dietary magnesium with cardiovascular disease, hypertension, diabetes, insulin, and carotid arterial wall thickness: The ARIC study (Atherosclerosis Risk in Communities Study). *Journal of Clinical Epidemiology*, volume 48, 927-940.

64. Dai Q, et al. (2007). The relation of magnesium and calcium intakes and a genetic polymorphism in the magnesium transporter to colorectal neoplasia risk. *American Journal of Clinical Nutrition*, volume 86, 743-751.

65. Larsson S, et al. (2005). Magnesium intake in relation to risk of colorectal cancer in women. *Journal of the American Medical Association*, volume 293, 86-89.

66. Larsson S, et al. (2005). Magnesium intake in relation to risk of colorectal cancer in women. *Journal of the American Medical Association*, volume 293, 86-89.

67. Larsson S, et al. (2005). Magnesium intake in relation to risk of colorectal cancer in women. *Journal of the American Medical Association*, volume 293, 86-89.

68. van den Brandt P, et al. (2007). Magnesium intake and colorectal cancer risk in the Netherlands Cohort Study. *British Journal of Cancer*, volume 96, 510-513.

69. Enbo M, et al. (2010). High dietary intake of magnesium may decrease risk of colorectal cancer in Japanese men. *Journal of Nutrition*, volume 140, 779-785.

70. Russo M, et al. (1997). Plasma selenium levels and the risk of colorectal adenomas. *Nutrition and Cancer*, volume 28(2), 125-129.

71. Knekt P, et al. (1998). Is low selenium status a risk factor for lung cancer? *American Journal of Epidemiology*, volume 148(10), 975-982.

72. Chu F, et al. (2004). Role of Se-dependent glutathione peroxidases in gastrointestinal inflammation and cancer. *Free Radical Biology and Medicine*, volume 36(12), 1481-1495.

73. Krukov G, et al. (2003). Characterization of mammalian selenoproteomes. *Science*, volume 300, 1439-1443.

74. Rotruck J, et al. (1973). Selenium: biochemical role as a component of glutathione peroxidase. *Science Magazine*, volume 179, 558-590.

75. Reeves M, Hoffmann P. (2009). The human selenoproteome: recent insights into functions and regulation. *Cellular and Molecular Life Sciences*, volume 66, 2457-2478.

76. Berry M, et al. (1991). Type I iodothyronine deiodinase is a selenocys-tein-containing enzyme. *Nature*, volume 349, 438-440.

77. Kohrei J. (2000). The deiodinase family: selenoenzymes regulating thyroid hormone availability and action. *Cellular and Molecular Life Sciences*, volume 57, 1853-1863.

78. Burk R, Hill K. (2009). Selenoprotein P-expression, functions and roles in mammals. *Biochimica et Biophysica Acta*, volume 1790, 1441-1447.

79. Thomson C, et al. (2005). The effect of selenium on thyroid status in a population with marginal selenium and iodine status. *British Journal of Nutrition*, volume 94, 962-968.

80. Bleys J, et al. (2008). Serum selenium levels and all-cause, cancer and cardiovascular mortality among US adults. *Archives of Internal Medicine*, volume 168, 404-410.

81. Akbaraly N, et al. (2005). Selenium and mortality in the elderly: results from the EVA study. *Clinical Chemistry*, volume 51, 2117-2123.

82. Ray A, et al. (2006). Low serum selenium and total carotenoids predict mortality among older women living in the community: the women's health and aging studies. *Journal of Nutrition*, volume 136, 172-176.

83. Zhuo H, et al. (2004). Selenium and lung cancer: a quantitative analysis of heterogeneity in the current epidemiological literature. *Cancer Epidemiology, Biomarkers & Prevention*, volume 13, 771-778.

84. Amaral A, et al. (2010). Selenium and bladder cancer risk: a meta-analysis. *Cancer Epidemiology, Biomarkers & Prevention*, volume 19(9), 2407-2415.

85. Etminan M, et al. (2005). Intake of selenium in the prevention of prostate cancer: a systematic review and meta-analysis. *Cancer Causes & Control*, volume 16, 1125-1131.

86. Brinkman M, et al. (2006). Are men with low selenium levels at increased risk of prostate cancer? *European Journal of Cancer*, volume 42, 2463-2471.

87. Clark L, et al. (1996). Effects of selenium supplementation for cancer prevention in patients with carcinoma of the skin. A randomized controlled trial. Nutritional Prevention of Cancer Study Group. *Journal of the American Medical Association*, volume 276, 1957-1963.

88. Duffield-Lillico A, et al. (2002). Baseline characteristics and the effect of selenium supplementation on cancer incidence in a randomized clinical trial: a summary report of the Nutritional Prevention of Cancer Trial. *Cancer Epidemiology, Biomarkers & Prevention,* volume 11, 630-639.

89. Maehira F, et al. (2002). Alterations of serum selenium concentrations in the acute phase of pathological conditions. *Clinica Chimica Acta*, volume 316, 137-146.

90. Helmersson J, et al. (2005). Serum selenium predicts levels of F2-isoprostanes and prostaglandin F2alpha in a 27 year follow-up study of Swedish men. *Free Radical Research*, volume 39(7), 763-770.

91. Angstwurm M, et al. (1999). Selenium replacement in patients with severe systemic inflammatory response syndrome improves clinical outcome. *Critical Care Medicine*, volume 27, 1807-1813.

92. Angstwurm M, et al. (2007). Selenium in Intensive Care (SIC): Results of a prospective randomized placebo-controlled, multiple-center study

in patients with severe systemic inflammatory response syndrome, sepsis and septic shock. *Critical Care Medicine*, volume 35, 118-126.

93. Barceloux D. (1999). Zinc. *Journal of Toxicology and Clinical Toxicology*, volume 37, 279-292.

94. Lonnerdal B. (2000). Dietary factors influencing zinc absorption. *Journal of Nutrition*, volume 130(5), 1378S-1383S.

95. Beattie J, Kwun I. (2004). Is zinc deficiency a risk factor for atherosclerosis? *British Journal of Nutrition*, volume 91(2), 177-181.

96. Vallee B, Falcuk K. (1993). The biochemical basis of zinc physiology. *Physiology Review*, volume 73(1), 79-118.

97. Uzzo R, et al. (2002). Zinc inhibits nuclear factor-kappa B activation and sensitizes prostate cancer cells to cytotoxic agents. *Clinical Cancer Research*, volume 8(11), 3579-3583.

98. Jeon K, et al. (2000). Thiol-reactive metal compounds inhibit NF-kappa B activation by blocking I kappa B kinase. *Journal of Immunology*, volume 164(11), 5981-5998.

99. Mocchegiani E, et al. (1998). Zinc, T-cell pathways, aging: role of metallothioneins. *Mechanisms of Ageing and Development*, volume 106, 183-204.

100. Wellinghausen N, et al. (1997). The immunobiology of zinc. *Immunology Today*, volume 18(11), 519-521.

101. Wapnir R. (2000). Zinc deficiency, malnutrition and the gastrointestinal tract. *Journal of Nutrition*, volume 130(suppl 5S), 1388S-1392S.

102. Mocchegiani E, et al. (2002). MtmRNA gene expression via IL-6 and glucocorticoids, as potential genetic marker of immunosenes-

cence: lessons from very old mice and humans. *Experimental Gerontology*, volume 37, 349-357.

103. Malavolta M, et al. (2006). Single and three-color flow cytometry assay for intracellular zinc ion availability in human lymphocytes with Zinpyr-1 and double immunofluorescence: Relationship with metallothioneins. *Cytometry Part A*, volume 69A, 1043-1053.

104. Bao B, et al. (2010). Zinc decreases C-reactive protein, lipid peroxidation, and inflammatory cytokines in elderly subjects: a potential implication of zinc as an atheroprotective agent. *American Journal of Clinical Nutrition*, volume 91, 1634-1641.

105. Kahmann L, et al. (2008). Zinc supplementation in the elderly reduces spontaneous inflammatory cytokine release and restores T cell functions. *Rejuvenation Research*, volume 11(1), 227-237.

106. Pourteymour F, et al. (2011). Effect of zinc supplementation on inflammatory markers in women with polycystic ovary syndrome. Shiraz E-Medical Journal, volume 12(1), http://semj.sums.ac.ir/vol12/jan2011/89007.htm.

107. Sutherland S, Browman G. (2001). Porphylaxis of oral mucositis in irradiated head-and-neck cancer patients: a proposed classification scheme of interventions and meta-analysis of randomized controlled trials. *International Journal of Radiation Oncology * Biology * Physics,* volume 49, 917-930.

108. Lin L, et al. (2006). Zinc supplementation to improve mucositis and dermatitis in patients after radiotherapy for head-and-neck cancers: a double-blind randomized study. *International Journal of Radiation Oncology * Biology * Physics,* volume 65, 745-750.

109. Lin L, et al. (2008). Effects of zinc supplementation on clinical outcomes in patients receiving radiotherapy for head and neck cancers: a double-blinded randomized study. *International Journal of Radiation Oncology * Biology * Physics*, volume 70(2), 368-373.

110. Dreno B, et al. (2005). Effect of zinc gluconate on propionibacterium acnes resistance to erythromycin in patients with inflammatory acne: in vitro and in vivo study. *European Journal of Dermatology*, volume 15(3), 152-155.

111. Dreno B, et al. (1989). Low doses of zinc gluconate for inflammatory acne. *Acta Dermato-Venereologica*, volume 69(6), 541-543.

112. Dreno B, et al. (2001). Multicenter randomized comparative double-blind controlled clinical trial of the safety and efficacy of zinc gluconate versus minocycline hydrocholoride in the treatment of inflammatory acne vulgaris. *Dermatology*, volume 203, 135-140.

113. Lips P. (2006). Vitamin D Physiology. *Progress in Biophysics and Molecular Biology*, volume 92, 4-8.

114. Peterson C, Heffernan M. (2008). Serum tumor necrosis factor-alpha concentrations are negatively correlated with serum 25(OH)D concentrations in healthy women. *Journal of Inflammation*, volume 5, 10-18.

115. Amer M, Qayyum R. (2012). Relation between serum 25-hydroxyvitamin D and C-reactive protein in asymptomatic adults (from the continuous National Health and Nutrition Examination Survey 2001 to 2006). *American Journal of Cardiology*, volume 109, 226-230.

116. Zhang Y, et al. (2012). Vitamin D inhibits monocyte/macrophage proinflammatory cytokine production by targeting MAPK phosphatase-1. *Journal of Immunology*, volume 188, 2127-2135.

117. Garland C, Garland F. (1980). Do sunlight and vitamin D reduced the likelihood of colon cancer? *International Journal of Epidemiology*, volume 9, 227-231.

118. Hanchette C, Schwartz G. (1992). Geographic patterns of prostate cancer mortality. Evidence for a protective effect of ultraviolet radiation. *Cancer*, volume 70, 2861-2869.

119. Giovannucci E. (2008). Vitamin D status and cancer incidence and mortality. *Advances in Experimental Medicine and Biology*, volume 624, 31-42.

120. Gorham E. et al (2005). Vitamin D and prevention of colorectal cancer. *Journal of Steroid Biochemistry and Molecular Biology*, volume 97, 179-184.

121. Gorham E. et al. (2007). Optimal vitamin D status for colorectal cancer prevention: a quantitative meta-analysis. *American Journal of Preventive Medicine*, volume 32, 210-216.

122. Wei M, et al. (2008). Vitamin D and prevention of colorectal adenoma: a meta-analysis. *Cancer Epidemiology, Biomarkers & Prevention*, volume 17, 2958-2969.

123. Garland C, et al. (1898). Serum 25-hydroxyvitamin D and colon cancer: eight-year prospective study. *Lancet*, volume 2, 1176-1178.

124. Garland C, et al. (2007). Vitamin D and prevention of breast cancer: pooled analysis. *Journal of Steroid Biochemistry and Molecular Biology*, volume 103, 708-711.

125. Ahonen M, et al. (2000). Porstate cancer risk and prediagnositc serum 25-hydroxyvitamin D levels. *Cancer Causes & Control*, volume 11, 847-852.

126. Bao B, et al. (2006). 1 alpha, 25-dihydorxyvitamin D3 suppresses interleukin-8-mediated prostate cancer cell angiogenesis. *Carcinogenesis*, volume 27, 1883-1893.

127. Criswell T, et al. (2003). Transcription factors activated in mammalian cells after clinically relevant doses of ionizing radiation. *Oncogene*, volume 22, 5813-5827.

128. Xu Y, et al. (2007). Suppression of ReIB-mediated manganese superoxide dismutase expression reveals a primary mechanism for radiosensitization effect of 1 alpha, 25-dihyroxyvitamin D(3) in prostate cancer cells. *Molecular Cancer Therapeutics*, volume 6, 2048-2056.

129. Krishnan A, et al. (2010). The role of vitamin D in cancer prevention and treatment. *Endocrinology and Metabolism Clinics of North America*, volume 39, 401-418.

130. Banach-Petrosky W, et al (2006). Vitamin D inhibits the formation of prostatic intraepithelial neoplasia in Nkx3.1;Pten mutant mice. *Clinical Cancer Research*, volume 12, 5895-5901.

131. Moreno J, et al. (2005). Regulation of prostaglandin metabolism by calcitriol attenuates growth stimulation in prostate cancer cells. *Cancer Research*, volume 65, 7917-7925.

132. Srinivas S, Feldman D. (2009). A phase II trial of calcitriol and naproxen in recurrent prostate cancer. *Anticancer Research*, volume 29, 3605-3610.

133. Nonn L, et al. (2006). Inhibition of p38 by vitamin D reduces interleukin-6 production in normal prostate cells via mitogen-activate protein kinase phosphatase 5: implications for prostate cancer prevention by vitamin D. *Cancer Research*, volume 66, 4516-4524.

134. Cerecetto H, Lopez G. (2007). Antioxidants derived from vitamin E: an overview. *Mini-Reviews in Medicinal Chemistry*, volume 7, 315-338.

135. "Peroxidation Mechanism." *Peroxidation Mechanism*. N.p., n.d. Web. 12 Oct. 2012. <http://www.cyberlipid.org/perox/oxid0006.htm>.

136. Burton G, Traber M. (1990). Vitamin E: antioxidant activity, bio-kinetics and bioavailability. *Annual Revue of Nutrition*, volume 10, 357-382.

137. Meydani M. (2001). Vitamin E and atherosclerosis: beyond prevention of LDL oxidation. *Journal of Nutrition*, volume 131, 366S-368S.

138. Iuliano L, et al. (2000). Radiolabeled native low-density lipoprotein injected into patients with carotid stenosis accumulates in macrophages of atherosclerotic plaque: effect of vitamin E supplementation. *Circulation*, volume 101, 1249-1254.

139. Cannon J, et al (1991). Acute phase response in exercise: Associations between vitamin E, cytokines and muscle proteolysis. *American Journal of Physiology*, volume 260, R1235-R1240.

140. Singh U, Devaraj S. (2007). Vitamin E: inflammation and athero-sclerosis. *Vitamins and Hormones*, volume 76, 519-549.

141. Devaraj S, et al. (2007). Effect of high-dose α-tocopherol supplementation on biomarkers of oxidative stress and inflammation and carotid atherosclerosis in patients with coronary artery disease. *American Journal of Clinical Nutrition*, volume 86, 1392-1398.

142. Devaraj S, et al. (1996). The effects of alpha-tocopherol supplementation on monocyte function: decreased lipid oxidation, interleukin

1 secretion, and monocyte adhesion to endothelium. *Journal of Clinical Investigation*, volume 98, 756-763.

143. Wu D, et al. (1999). Effect of vitamin E on human aortic endothelial cell production of chemokines and adhesion to monocytes. *Atherosclerosis*, volume 147, 297-307.

144. Freedman J, et al. (1996). Alpha-tocopherol inhibits aggregation of human platelets by a protein kinase C-dependent mechanism. *Circulation*, volume 94, 2434-2440.

145. Gey K, et al. (1993). Increased risk of cardiovascular disease at suboptimal plasma concentrations of essential antioxidants: an epidemiological update with special attention to carotene and vitamin C. *American Journal of Clinical Nutrition*, volume 57(suppl), 787S-797S.

146. Rimm E, et al. (1993). Vitamin E consumption and the risk of coronary heart disease in men. *New England Journal of Medicine*, volume 328, 1450-1456.

147. Stampfer M, et al. (1993). Vitamin E consumption and the risk of coronary disease in women. *New England Journal of Medicine*, volume 328, 1444-1449.

148. Losonczy K, et al. (1996). Vitamin E and vitamin C supplement use and risk of all-cause and coronary heart disease mortality in older persons: the Established Populations for Epidemiologic Studies of the Elderly. *American Journal of Clinical Nutrition*, volume 64, 190-196.

149. Stephens N, et al. (1996). Randomized controlled trial of vitamin E in patients with coronary disease: Cambridge Heart Antioxidant Study (CHAOS). *Lancet*, volume 347, 781-786.

150. Salonen J, et al. (2000). Antioxidant Supplementation in Athero-sclerosis (ASAP) study: a randomized trial of the effect of Vitamins E and C on 3-year progression of carotid atherosclerosis. *Journal of Internal Medicine*, volume 248, 377-386.

151. Blot W, et al. (1993). Nutrition intervention trials in Linxian, China: supplementation with specific vitamin/mineral combinations, cancer incidence, and disease-specific mortality in the general population. *Journal of the National Cancer Institute*, volume 85, 1483-1492.

152. The Alpha-Tocopherol, Beta-Carotene Cancer Prevention Study Group. (1994). The effect of vitamin E and beta-carotene on the incidence of lung cancer and other cancers in male smokers. *New England Journal of Medicine*, volume 330, 1029-1035.

153. Comstock G, et al. (1992). Serum retinol, beta-carotene, vitamin E and selenium as related to subsequent cancer of specific sites. *American Journal of Epidemiology*, volume 135, 115-121.

154. Bostik R, et al. (1993). Reduced risk of colon cancer with high intake of vitamin E: the Iowa Women's Health Study. *Cancer Research*, volume 53, 4230-4237.

155. Tsao R. (2010). Chemistry and biochemistry of dietary polyphenols. *Nutrients*, volume 2, 1231-1246.

156. Renaud S, Lorgeril M. (1992). Wine, alcohol, platelets, and the French paradox for coronary heart disease. *Lancet*, volume 339, 1523-1526.

157. Ignatowicz E, Dubowska W. (2001). Resveratrol, a natural chemo-preventive agent against degenerative disease. *Polish Journal of Pharmacology*, volume 53, 557-569.

158. Das S, Das D. (2007). Anti-inflammatory responses of resveratrol. *Inflammation and Allergy-Drug Targets*, volume 6, 168-173.

159. Martinez J, Moreno J. (2000). Effect of resveratrol, a natural polyphenolic compound, on reactive oxygen species and prostaglandin production. *Biochemical Pharmacology*, volume 59, 865-870.

160. Birrell M, et al. (2005). Resveratrol, an extract of red wine, inhibits lipopolysaccharide induced airway neutrophilia and inflammatory mediators through an NF-κB-independent mechanism. *FASEB Journal*, volume 19, 840-841.

161. Manna S, et al. (2000). Resveratrol suppresses TNF-induced acdtivation of nuclear transcription factors NF-kappa B, activator protein-1, and apoptosis: potential role of reactive oxygen intermediates and lipid peroxidation. *Journal of Immunology*, volume 164, 6509-6519.

162. Yu L, et al. (2008). Resveratrol inhibits tumor necrosis factor-[alpha]-mediated matrix metalloproteinase-9 expression and invasion of human hepatocellular carcinoma cells. *Biomedical Pharmacotherapy*, volume 62, 366-372.

163. Zhu J, et al. (2008). Anti-inflammatory effect of resveratrol on TNF-alpha-induced MCP-1 expression in adipocytes. *Biochemical and Biophysical Research Communications*, volume 369, 471-477.

164. Szewczuk L, et al. (2004). Resveratrol is a peroxidase-mediated inactivator of COX-1 but not COX-2. *Journal of Biological Chemistry*, volume 279, 22727-22737.

165. Subbaramaiah K, et al. (1998). Resveratrol inhibits cycloocygenase-2 transcription and activity in phorbol ester-treated human mammary

epithelial cells. *Journal of Biological Chemistry*, volume 273, 21875-21882.

166. Khanduja K, et al. (2004). Resveratrol inhibits N-nitrosodiethyl-amine-induced ornithine decarboxylase and cyclooxygenase in mice. *Journal of Nutritional Science and Vitaminology*, volume 50, 61-65.

167. Varraso R, et al. (2007). Prospective study of dietary patterns and chronic obstructive pulmonary disease among US women. *American Journal of Clinical Nutrition*, volume 86, 488-495.

168. Wickens K, et al. (2005). Fast foods—are they a risk factor for asthma? *Allergy*, volume 60, 1537-1541.

169. Shaheen S, et al. (2001). Dietary antioxidants and asthma in adults. *American Journal of Respiratory and Critical Care Medicine*, volume 164, 1823-1828.

170. Liu J, et al. (2003). Inhibition of cyclic strain-induced endothelin-1 gene expression by resveratrol. *Hypertension*, volume 42, 1198-1205.

171. Zou J, et al. (2003). Effect of red wine and wine polyphenol resvera-trol on endothelial function in hypercholesterolemic rabbits. *International Journal of Molecular Medicine*, volume 11, 317-320.

172. Fremont L, et al. (1999). Antioxidant activity of resveratrol and alcohol-free wine polyphenols related to LDL oxidation and polyunsatu-rated fatty acids. *Life Sciences*, volume 64, 2511-2521.

173. Leighton F, et al. (1999). Plasma polyphenols and antioxidants, oxidative DNA damage and endothelial function in diet and wine intervention study in humans. *Drugs Under Experimental and Clinical Research*, volume 15, 133-141.

174. Bhavnani B, et al. (2001). Comparison of the antioxidant effects of equine estrogens, red wine components, vitamin E, and probucol on low-density lipoprotein oxidation in postmenopausal women. *Menopause*, volume 8, 408-419.

175. Godichaud S, et al. (2000). Deactivation of cultured human liver myofibroblasts by trans-resveratrol, a grapevine-derived polyphenol. *Hepatology*, volume 31, 922-931.

176. Pace-Asciak C, et al. (1995). The red wine phenolics trans-resveratrol and quercetin block human platelet aggregation and eicosanoid synthesis: implications for protection against coronary heart disease. *Clinica Chimica Acta*, volume 31, 207-219.

177. Dobrydneva Y, et al. (1999). Trans-resveratrol inhibits calcium influx in thrombin-stimulated human platelets. *British Journal of Pharmacology*, volume 128, 149-157.

178. Pendurthi U, et al. (1999). Resveratrol, a polyphenolic compound found in wine, inhibits tissue factor expression in vascular cells. *Arteriosclerosis, Thrombosis, and Vascular Biology*, volume 19, 419-426.

179. Pendurthi U, et al. (2002). Mechanism of resveratrol-mediated suppression of tissue factor gene expression. *Journal of Thrombosis and Haemostasis*, volume 87, 155-162.

180. Zou J, et al. (1999). Suppression of mitogenesis and regulation of cell cycle traverse by resveratrol in cultured smooth muscle cells. *International Journal of Oncology*, volume 15, 647-651.

181. Mnjoyan Z, Fujise K. (2003). Profound negative regulatory effects by resveratrol on vascular smooth muscle cells: a role of p53-p21

WAF1/CIP1 pathway. *Biochemical and Biophysical Research Communications*, volume 311, 546-552.

182. Clement M, et al. (1998). Chemopreventive agent resveratrol, a natural product derived from grapes, triggers CD95 signaling-dependent apoptosis in human tumor cells. *Blood*, volume 92, 996-1002.

183. Huang C, et al. (1999). Resveratrol suppresses cell transformation and induces apoptosis through a p53-dependent pathway. *Carcinogenesis*, volume 20, 237-242.

184. Ferrazzano G, et al. (2011). Plant polyphenols and their anti-cariogenic properties: a review. *Molecules*, volume 16, 1486-1507.

185. Cal C, et al. (2003). Resveratrol and cancer: chemoprevention, apoptosis, and chemoimmunosensitizing activities. *Current Medicinal Chemistry – Anti-Cancer Agents*, volume 3, 77-93.

186. Hsieh T, et al. (1999). Cell cycle effects and control of gene expression by resveratrol in human breast carcinoma cell lines with different metastatic potentials. *International Journal of Oncology*, volume 15, 245-252.

187. Jang M, et al. (1997). Cancer chemopreventive activity of resveratrol, a natural product derived from grapes. *Science*, volume 275, 218-220.

188. Garvin S, et al. (2006). Resveratrol induces apoptosis and inhibits angiogenesis in human breast cancer xenografts in vivo. *Cancer Letters*, volume 231, 113-122.

189. Wietzke J, Welsh J. (2003). Phytoestrogen regulation of a Vitamin D_3 receptor promoter and 1,25-dihydroxyvitamin D_3 actions in human breast cancer cells. *Journal of Steroid Biochemistry and Molecular Biology*, volume 84, 149-157.

190. Rimsza L, et al. (2003). Endothelial stimulation by small lympho-cytic lymphoma correlates with secreted levels of basic fibroblastic growth factor. *British Journal of Haematology*, volume 120, 753-758.

191. Ferry-Dumazet H, et al. (2002). Resveratrol inhibits the growth and induces the apoptosis of both normal and leukemic hematopoietic cells. *Carcinogenesis*, volume 23, 1327-1333.

192. Kang H, et al. (2011). Antiproliferation and redifferentiation in thy-roid cancer cell lines by polyphenol phytochemicals. *Journal of Korean Medical Science*, volume 26, 893-899.

193. Mitchell S, et al. (1999). Differential effects on growth, cell cycle arrest and induction of apoptosis by resveratrol in human prostate cancer cell lines. *Experimental Cell Research*, volume 249, 109-115.

194. Hsieh T, Wu J. (2000). Grape-derived chemopreventive agent resve-ratrol decreases prostate-specific antigen (PSA) expression in LNCaP cells by an androgen receptor (AR)-independent mechanism. *Anti-cancer Research*, volume 20, 225-228.

195. Kaiberlein M, et al. (1999). The SIR2/3/4 complex and SIR2 alone promote longevity in *Saccharomyces cerevisiae* by two different mecha-nisms. *Genes & Development*, volume 13, 2570-2580.

196. Lin S, et al. (2000). Requirement of NAD and SIR2 for life-span extension by calorie restriction in *Saccharomyces cerevisiae*. *Science*, vol-ume 289, 2126-2128.

197. Howitz K, et al. (2003). Small molecule activators of sirtuins extend *Saccharomyces cerevisiae* lifespan. *Nature*, volume 425, 191-196.

198. Wood J, et al. (2004). Sirtuin activators mimic caloric restriction and delay ageing in metazoans. *Nature*, volume 430, 686-689.

199. Valenzano D, et al. (2006). Resveratrol prolongs lifespan and retards the onset of age-related markers in a short-lived vertebrate. *Current Biology*, volume 16, 296-300.

200. Baur J, et al. (2006). Resveratrol improves health and survival of mice on a high-calorie diet. *Nature*, volume 444, 337-342.

201. Chandrashekara K, Shakarad M. (2011). Aloe vera or resveratrol supplementation in larval diet delays adult aging in the fruit fly, *Drosophila melanogaster. Journals of Gerontology, Series A, Biological Sciences and Medical Sciences*, volume 66, 965-971.

202. Timmers S, et al. (2011). Calorie restriction-like effects of 30 days of resveratrol supplementation on energy metabolism and metabolic profile in obese humans. *Cell Metabolism*, volume 14, 612-622.

203. Maheshwari R, et al. (2006). Multiple biological activities of curcumin: a short review. *Life Sciences*, volume 78, 2081-2087.

204. Shukla P, et al. (2003). Protective effect of curcumin against lead neurotoxicity in rat. *Human & Experimental Toxicology*, volume 22, 653-658.

205. Manjunatha H, Srinivasan K. (2007). Hypolipidemic and antioxidant effects of curcumin and capsaicin in high-gat-fed rats. *Canadian Journal of Physiology and Pharmacology*, volume 85, 588-596.

206. Chan W, Wu H. (2006). Protective effects of curcumin on methylglyoxal-induced oxidative DNA damage and cell injury in human mononuclear cells. *Acta Pharmacologica Sinica*, volume 27, 1192-1198.

207. DiSilvestro R. "Curcumin Extract Lowers Triglycerides, Boosts Antioxidant Activity: Ohio State Study" *Ohio State University Extension.*

Ed. Mauricio Espinoza. The Ohio State University Extension, 10 May 2012. Web. 19 Aug. 2012. <http://geauga.osu.edu/news-releases/archives/2012/may/curcumin-extract-lowers-triglycerides-boosts-antioxidant-activity-ohio-state-study>.

208. Mahfouz M, et al. (2009). Curcumin prevents the oxidation and lipid modification of LDL and its inhibition of prostacyclin generation by endothelial cells in culture. *Prostaglandins and Other Lipid Mediators*, volume 90, 13-20.

209. Dhillon N, et al. (2006). Phase II trial of curcumin (diferuloyl methane), an NF-κB inhibitor, in patients with advanced pancreatic cancer. *Journal of Clinical Oncology*, volume 24, 14151.

210. Vadhan-Raj, S., et al. (2007). Curcumin downregulates NF-κB and related genes in patients with multiple myeloma: results of a phase 1/2 study. American Society of Hematology Annual Meeting.

211. Jobin C, et al. (1999). Curcumin blocks cytokine-mediated ND-kappa B activation and proinflammatory gene expression by inhibiting inhibitory factor I-kappa B kinase activity. *Journal of Immunology*, volume 163, 3474-3483.

212. Surh Y, et al. (2001). Molecular mechanisms underlying chemopreventive activities of anti-inflammatory phytochemicals: down-regulation of COX-2 and iNOS through suppression of NF-kappa B activation. *Mutation Research*, volume 480, 243-268.

213. Kunnumakkara A, et al. (2007). Curcumin potentiates antitumor activity of gemcitabine in an orthotopic model of pancreatic cancer through suppression of proliferation, angiogenesis, and inhibition of nuclear factor-kappa B-related gene products. *Cancer Research*, volume 67, 3853-3861.

214. Lin Y, et al. (2007). Curcumin inhibits tumor growth and angiogenesis in ovarian carcinoma by targeting the nuclear factor-kappa B pathway. *Clinical Cancer Research*, volume 13, 3423-3430.

215. Wang X, et al. (2006). Curcumin inhibits neurotensin-mediated interleukin-8 production and migration of HCT116 human colon cancer cells. *Clinical Cancer Research*, volume 12, 5346-5355.

216. Aggarwal B, et al. (2005). Curcumin suppresses the paclitaxel-induced nuclear factor-κB pathway in breast cancer cells and inhibits lung metastasis of human breast cancer in nude mice. *Clinical Cancer Research*, volume 11, 7490-7498.

217. Cruz-Correa M, et al. (2006). Combination treatment with curcumin and quercetin of adenomas in familial adenomatous polyposis. *Clinical Gastroenterology and Hepatology*, volume 4, 1035-1038.

218. Park J, Conteas C. (2010). Anti-carcinogenic properties of curcumin on colorectal cancer. *World Journal of Gastrointestinal Oncology*, volume 2, 169-176.

219. Formica J, Regelson W. (1995). Review of the biology of quercetin and related bioflavonoids. *Food and Chemical Toxicology*, volume 33, 1061-1080.

220. Erlund I. (2004). Review of the flavonoids quercetin, hesperetin, and naringenin. Dietary sources, bioactivities, bioavailability, and epidemiology. *Nutrition Research*, volume 24, 851-874.

221. Chi Y, et al. (2001). Effects of naturally occurring prenylated flavonoids on arachidonic acid metabolizing enzymes: cyclooxygenases and lipoxygenases. *Biochemical Pharmacology*, volume 62, 1185-1191.

222. Min Y, et al. (2007). Quercetin inhibits expression of inflammatory cytokines through attenuation of NF-κB and p38 MAPK in HMC-1 human mast cell line. *Inflammation Research*, volume 56, 210-215.

223. Ruiz P, et al. (2007). Quercetin inhibits TNF-induced NF-κB transcription factor recruitment to proinflammatory gene promoters in murine intestinal epithelial cells. *Journal of Nutrition*, volume 137, 1206-1215.

224. Avila M, et al. (1994). Quercetin mediates the down-regulation of mutant p53 in the human breast cancer cell line, MDA-MB468. *Cancer Research*, volume 54, 2424-2428.

225. Avila M, et al. (1996). Quercetin as a modulator of the cellular neoplastic phenotype. *Advances in Experimental Medicine and Biology*, volume 401, 101-110.

226. Yoshida M, et al. (1992). Quercetin arrest human leukemic T-cells in late G1 phase of the cell cycle. *Cancer Research*, volume 52, 6676-6681.

227. Yoshida M, et al. (1990). The effect of quercetin on cell cycle progression and growth of human gastric cancer cells. *Federation of European Biochemical Societies Letters*, volume 260, 10-13.

228. Aalinkeel R, et al. (2008). The dietary bioflavonoid, quercetin, selectively induces apoptosis of prostate cancer cells by down-regulating the expression of heat shock protein 90. *The Prostate*, volume 68, 1773-1789.

229. Borska S, et al. (2010). Antiproliferative and pro-apoptotic effects of quercetin on human pancreatic carcinoma cell lines EPP85-181P and EPP85-181RDB. *Folia Histochemica et Cytobiologica*, volume 48, 222-229.

230. Kyle J, et al. (2009). Dietary flavonoid intake and colorectal cancer: a case-control study. *British Journal of Nutrition*, volume 103, 429-436.

231. Knekt P, et al. (2002). Flavonoid intake and risk of chronic diseases. *American Journal of Clinical Nutrition*, volume 76, 560-568.

232. De Stefani E, et al. (1999). Dietary antioxidants and lung cancer risk: a case-control study in Uruguay. *Nutrition and Cancer*, volume 34, 100-110.

233. Nöthlings U, et al. (2008). A food pattern that is predictive of flavonol intake and risk of pancreatic cancer. *American Journal of Clinical Nutrition*, volume 88, 1653-1662.

234. Bobe G, et al. (2008). Flavonoid intake and risk of pancreatic cancer in male smokers. *Cancer Epidemiology, Biomarkers & Prevention*, volume 17, 553-562.

235. Wilson R, et al. (2009). Fish, vitamin D, and flavonoids in relation to renal cell cancer among smokers. *American Journal of Epidemiology*, volume 170, 717-729.

236. Lee S, et al. (2009). Inhibitory effects of flavonoids on TNF-alpha-induced IL-8 gene expression in HEK 293 cells. *Biochemistry and Molecular Biology Reports*, volume 42, 265-270.

237. Kempuraj D, et al. (2005). Flavonols inhibit proinflammatory mediator release, intracellular calcium ion levels and protein kinase C theta phosphorylation in human mast cells. *British Journal of Pharmacology*, volume 145, 934-944.

238. Comalada M, et al. (2006). Inhibition of pro-inflammatory markers in primary bone marrow-derived mouse macrophages by naturally

occurring flavonoids: analysis of the structure-activity relationship. *Biochemical Pharmacology*, volume 72, 1010-1021.

239. Sharma V, et al. (2007). Modulation of interleukin-1 beta mediated inflammatory response in human astrocytes by flavonoids: implications in neuroprotection. *Brain Research Bulletin*, volume 73, 55-63.

240. Ying B, et al. (2009). Quercetin inhibits IL-1 beta-induced ICAM-1 expression in pulmonary epithelial cell line A549 through the MAPK pathways. *Molecular Biology Reports*, volume 36, 1825-1832.

241. O'Reilly J, et al. (2000). Flavonoids protect against oxidative damage to LDL in vitro: use in selection of a flavonoid rich diet and relevance to LDL oxidation resistance ex vivo? *Free Radical Research*, volume 33, 419-426.

242. O'Reilly J, et al. (2000). Flavonoids protect against oxidative damage to LDL in vitro: use in selection of a flavonoid rich diet and relevance to LDL oxidation resistance ex viv? *Free Radical Research*, volume 33, 419-426.

243. Ozgova S, et al. (2003). Different antioxidant effects of polyphenols on lipid peroxidation and hydroxyl radicals in the NADPH-FE-ascorbate- and Fe-microsomal systems. *Biochemical Pharmacology*, volume 66, 1127-1285.

244. Lopez-Lopez G, et al. (2004). Nitric Oxide NO; scavenging and NO protecting effects of quercetin and their biological significance in vascular smooth muscle. *Molecular Pharmacology*, volume 65, 851-859.

245. Appel L, et al. (1997). A clinical trial of the effects of dietary patterns on blood pressure. *New England Journal of Medicine*, volume 33, 1117-1124.

246. Duarte J, et al. (1993). Vasodilator effects of quercetin in isolated rate vascular smooth muscle. *European Journal of Pharmacology*, volume 239, 1-7.

247. Duarte J, et al. (2001). Antihypertensive effects of the flavonoid quercetin in spontaneously hypertensive rats. *British Journal of Pharmacology*, volume 133, 117-124.

248. Edwards R, et al. (2007). Quercetin reduces blood pressure in hypertensive subjects. *Journal of Nutrition*, volume 137, 2405-2411.

249. Huang Y, et al. (1999). Effects of luteolin and quercetin: Inhibitors of tyrosine kinase, on cell growth and metastasis-associated properties in A431 cells over-expressing epidermal growth fact receptor. *British Journal of Pharmacology*, volume 28, 999-1010.

250. Gryglewski R, et al (1987). On the mechanism of antithrombotic action of flavonoids. *Biochemical Pharmacology*, volume 36, 317-322.

251. Hubbard G, et al. (2004). Ingestion of quercetin inhibits platelet aggregation and essential components of the collagen-stimulated platelet activation pathway in humans. *Journal of Thrombosis and Haemostasis*, volume 2, 2138-2145.

252. Stein J, et al. (1999). Purple grape juice improves endothelial function and reduces the susceptibility of LDL cholesterol to oxidation in patients with coronary artery disease. *Circulation*, volume 100, 1050-1055.

253. Rendig S, et al. (2001). Effects of red wine, alcohol, and quercetin on coronary reisstance and conductance arteries. *Journal of Cardiovascular Pharmaoclogy*, volume 38, 219-227.

254. Nettleton J. (1995). *Omega-3 Fatty Acid and Health*. New York: Chapman & Hall, pp 21-30.

255. Wang Y, et al. (1990). Omega-3 fatty acid in Lake Superior fish. *Journal of Food Science*, volume 55, 71-73.

256. Spiller G. (1996). *Lipid in Human Nutrition Handbook, Manuals etc.* Boca Raton: CRS Press, Inc., p 54.

257. Chan E, Cho L. (2009). What can we expect from omega-3 fatty acids? *Cleveland Clinic Journal of Medicine*, volume 76, 245-251.

258. Lee J, et al. (2009). Omega-3 fatty acids: cardiovascular benefits, sources and sustainability. *Nature Reviews Cardiology*, volume 6, 753-758.

259. Simopoulos A. (2002). The importance of the ratio of omega-6/omega-3 essential fatty acids. *Biomedical Pharmacotherapy*, volume 56, 365-379.

260. Browning L, et al. (2006). The impact of long chain n-3 polyunsaturated fatty acid supplementation on inflammation, insulin sensitivity and CVD risk in a group of overweight women with an inflammatory phenotype. *Diabetes, Obesity and Metabolism*, volume 9, 70-80.

261. Bloomer R, et al. (2009). Effect of eicosapentaenoic and docosahexaenoic acid on resting and exercise-induced inflammatory and oxidative stress biomarkers: a randomized, placebo-controlled, cross-over study. *Lipids in Health and Disease*, volume 8, 36-48.

262. Tsitouras P, et al. (2008). High omega-3 fat intake improves insulin sensitivity and reduces CRP and IL-6, but does not affect other endocrine axes in healthy older adults. *Hormone and Metabolic Research*, volume 40, 199-205.

263. Morledge M, et al. (2011). Omega-3 FAs reduce serum C-reactive protein concentration. *Clinical Lipidology*, volume 6, 723-729

264. Moghadam M, et al. (2012). Efficacy of omega-3 fatty acid supplementation on serum levels of tumour necrosis factor-alpha, C-reactive protein and interleukin-2 in type 2 diabetes mellitus patients. *Singapore Medical Journal*, volume 53, 615-619.

265. Zhao Y, et al. (2009). Effects of n-3 polyunsaturated fatty acid therapy on plasma inflammatory markers and N-terminal pro-brain natriuretic peptide in elderly patients with chronic heart failure. *The Journal of International Medical Research*, volume 37, 1831-1841.

266. Caughey G, et al. (1996). The effect on human tumor necrosis factor alpha and interleukin 1 beta production of diets enriched in n-3 fatty acids from vegetable oil or fish oil. *American Journal of Clinical Nutrition*, volume 63, 116-122.

267. De Caterina R, Libby P. (1996). Control of endothelial leukocyte adhesion molecules by fatty acids. *Lipids*, volume 31, S57-S63.

268. De Caterina R, et al. (2000). Fatty acid modulation of endothelial activation. *American Journal of Clinical Nutrition*, volume 21, 213S-223S.

269. Yang Y, et al. (2012). Effects of n-3 PUFA supplementation on plasma soluble adhesion molecules: a meta-analysis of randomized controlled trials. *American Journal of Clinical Nutrition*, volume 95, 972-980.

270. Smith S Jr, et al. (2011). AHA/ACCF secondary prevention and risk reduction therapy for patients with coronary and other

atherosclerotic vascular disease: 2011 update. *Circulation*, volume 124, 2458-2473.

271. Kromhout D, et al. (1985). The inverse relation between fish consumption and 20-year mortality from coronary heart disease. *New England Journal of Medicine*, volume 312, 1205-1209.

272. Dolecek T, et al. (1991). Dietary polyunsaturated fatty acids and mortality in the Multiple Risk Factor Intervention Trial (MRFIT). *World Review Of Nutrition and Dietetics*, volume 66, 205-216.

273. Kromhout D, et al. (1995). The protective effect of a small amount of fish on coronary heart disease mortality in an elderly population. *International Journal of Epidemiology*, volume 24, 340-345.

274. Hu F, et al. (2002). Fish and omega-3 fatty acid intake and risk of coronary heart disease in women. *Journal of the American Medical Association*, volume 287, 1815-1821.

275. He K, et al. (2004). Accumulated evidence on fish consumption and coronary heart disease mortality: a meta-analysis of cohort studies. *Circulation*, volume 109, 2705-2711.

276. Burr M, et al. (1989). Effects of changes in fat, fish, and fibre intakes on death and myocardial reinfarction: Diet and Reinfarction Trial (DART). *Lancet*, volume 334, 757-761.

277. Singh R, et al. (1997). Randomized, double-blind, placebo-controlled trial of fish oil and mustard oil in patients with suspected acute myocardial infarction: the Indian experiment of infarct survival-4. *Cardiovascular Drugs and Therapy*, volume 11, 485-491.

278. Gruppo Italioano per lo Studio della Spravvievenza nell'Infarto miocardioco. (1999). Dietary supplementation with n-3 polyunsaturated

fatty acids and vitamin E after myocardial infarction: results of the GISSI-Prevenzione trial. *Lancet*, volume 354, 447-455.

279. von Schacky C, et al. (1999). The effect of dietary omega-3 fatty acids on coronary atherosclerosis: a randomized, double-blind, placebo-controlled trial. *Annals of Internal Medicine*, volume 130, 554-562.

280. Eritsland J, et al. (1996). Effect of dietary supplementation with n-3 fatty acids on coronary artery bypass graft patency. *American Journal of Cardiology*, volume 77, 31-36.

281. Appel L, et al. (1993). Does supplementation of diet with 'fish oil' reduce blood pressure? A meta-analysis of controlled clinical trials. *Archives of Internal Medicine*, volume 153, 1429-1438.

282. Morris M, et al. (1993). Does fish oil lower blood pressure? A meta-analysis of controlled trials. *Circulation*, volume 88, 523-533.

283. Knapp H. (1997). Dietary fatty acids in human thrombosis and hemostasis. *American Journal of Clinical Nutrition*, volume 65, 1687S-1698S.

284. Mori T, et al. (1997). Interactions between dietary fat, fish, and fish oils and their effects on platelet function in men at risk of cardiovascular disease. *Arteriosclerosis, Thrombosis, and Vascular Biology*, volume 17, 279-286.

285. Barcelli U, et al. (1985). Enhancing effect of dietary supplementation with omega-3 fatty acids on plasma fibrinolysis in normal subjects. *Thrombosis Research*, volume 39, 307-312.

286. Siasos G, et al. (2011). Effects of omega-3 fatty acids on endothelial function, arterial wall properties, inflammatory and fibrinolytic

status in smokers: a cross over study. *International Journal of Cardiology*, e-published November 21.

287. Harris W. (1997). n-3 Fatty acids and serum lipoproteins: human studies. *American Journal of Clinical Nutrition*, volume 65, 1645S-1654S.

288. Koski R. (2008). Omega-3-acid ethyl esters (Lovaza) for severe hypertriglyceridemia. *Pharmacy and Therapeutics*, volume 33, 271-303.

289. Gago-Dominguez M, et al. (2003). Opposing effects of dietary n-3 and n-6 fatty acids on mammary carcinogenesis: The Singapore Chinese Heatlh Study. *British Journal of Cancer*, volume 89, 1686-1692.

290. Thiebaut A, et al. (2009). Dietary intakes of omega-6 and omega-3 polyunsaturated fatty acids and the risk of breast cancer. *International Journal of Cancer*, volume 124, 924-931.

291. Murff H, et al. (2011). Dietary polyunsaturated fatty acids and breast cancer risk in Chinese women: a prospective cohort study. *International Journal of Cancer*, volume 128, 1434-1441.

292. Chajes V, et al. (2012). ω-3 and ω-6 polyunsaturated fatty acid intakes and the risk of breast cancer in Mexican women: impact of obesity status. *Cancer Epidemiology, Biomarkers & Prevention*, volume 21, 319-326.

293. Rubin P, Millison K. (2007). Pharmacotherapy of disease mediated by 5-lipoxygenase pathway eicosanoids. *Prostaglandins and Other Lipid Mediators*, volume 83, 188-197.

294. Soumaoro L, et al. (2006). Expression of 5-lipoxygenase in human colorectal cancer. *World Journal of Gastroenterology*, volume 12, 6355-6360.

295. Ghosh J, Myers C. (1997). Arachidonic acid stimulates prostate cancer cell growth: critical role of 5-lipoxygenase. *Biochemical and Biophysical Research Communications*, volume 235, 418-423.

296. Tong W, et al. (2005). LTB4 stimulates growth of human pancreatic cancer cells via MAPK and PI-3 kinase pathways. *Biochemical and Biophysical Research Communications,* volume 335, 949-956.

297. Jiang W, et al. (2003). Levels of expression of lipoxygenases and cyclooxygenases-2 in human breast cancer. *Prostaglandins, Leukotrienes and Essential Fatty Acids*, volume 69, 275-281.

298. Wang J, et al. (2008). 5-lipoxygenase and 5-liposygenase-activating protein gene polymorphisms, dietary linoleic acid and risk for breast cancer. *Cancer Epidemiology, Biomarkers & Prevention*, volume 17, 2748-2754.

299. Bower J, et al. (2006). Fatigue in long-term breast carcinoma survivors: a longitudinal investigation. *Cancer*, volume 106, 751-758.

300. Lee B, et al. (2004). A cytokine-based neuroimmunologic mechanism of cancer-related symptoms. *Neuroimmunomodulation*, volume 11, 279-292.

301. Schubert C, et al. (2007). The association between fatigue and inflammatory marker levels in cancer patients: a quantitative review. *Brain, Behavior, and Immunity*, volume 21, 413-427.

302. Bower J, et al. (2009). Inflammatory biomarkers and fatigue during radiation therapy for breast and prostate cancer. *Clinical Cancer Research*, volume 15, 5534-5540.

303. Ferrucci L, et al. (2006). Relationship of plasma polyunsaturated fatty acids to circulating inflammatory markers. *Journal of Clinical Endocrinology & Metabolism*, volume 91, 439-446.

304. Kalogeropoulos N, et al. (2010). Unsaturated fatty acids are inversely associated and n-6/n-3 ratios are positively related to inflammation and coagulation markers in plasma of apparently healthy adults. *Clinica Chimica Acta*, volume 411, 584-591.

305. Alfano C, et al. (2012). Fatigue, inflammation, and ω-3 and ω-6 fatty acid intake among breast cancer survivors. *Journal of Clinical Oncology*, volume 30, 1280-1287.

306. Pearce M, Dayton S. (1971). Incidence of cancer in men on a diet high in polyunsaturated fat. *Lancet*, volume 1, 464-467.

307. Sasazuki S, et al. (2011). Intake of n-3 and n-6 polyunsaturated fatty acids and development of colorectal cancer by subsite: Japan Public Health Center-based prospective study. *International Journal of Cancer*, volume 129, 1718-1729.

308. Geelan A, et al. (2007). Fish consumption, n-3 fatty acids, and colorectal cancer: a meta-analysis of prospective cohort studies. *American Journal of Epidemiology*, volume 166, 1116-1125.

309. Kim S, et al. (2010). Intake of polyunsaturated fatty acids and distal large bowel cancer risk in whites and African Americans. *American Journal of Epidemiology*, volume 171, 969-979

310. Pot G, et al. (2008). Opposing associations of serum n-3 and n-6 polyunsaturated fatty acids with colorectal adenoma risk: an endoscopy-based case-control study. *International Journal of Cancer*, volume 123, 1974-1977.

311. West N, et al. (2010). Eicosapentaenoic acid reduces rectal polyp number and size in familial adenomatous polyposis. *Gut*, volume 59, 918-925.

312. Calviello G, et al. (2005). Docosahexaenoic acid enhances the susceptibility of human colorectal cancer cells to 5-fluorouracil. *Cancer Chemotherapy and Pharmacology*, volume 55, 12-20.

313. Jordan A, Stein J. (2003). Effect of an omega-3 fatty acid containing lipid emulsion alone and in combination with 5-fluorouracil (5-FU) on growth of the colon cancer cell line Caco-2. *European Journal of Nutrition,* volume 42, 324-331.

314. Taussig S, Batkin S. (1988). Bromelain, the enzyme complex of pineapple (Ananas comosus) and its clinical application. An update. *Journal of Ethnopharmacology*, volume 22, 191-203.

315. Maurer H. (2001). Bromelain: biochemistry, pharmacology and medical use. *Cellular and Molecular Life Sciences*, volume 58, 1234-1245.

316. "Bromelain." *Bromelain*. N.p., 06 Apr. 2011. Web. 28 Dec. 2012. <http://www.cancer.org/treatment/treatmentsandsideeffects/complementaryandalternativemedicine/herbsvitaminsandminerals/bromelain>.

317. Desser L, et al. (1994). Proteolytic enzymes and amylase induce cytokine production in human peripheral blood mononuclear cells in vitro. *Cancer Biotherapy and Radiopharmaceuticals*, volume 9, 253-263.

318. Engwerda C, et al. (2001). Bromelain activates murine macrophages and natural killer cells in vitro. *Cell Immunology*, volume 210, 5-10.

319. Barth H, et al. (2005). In vitro study on the immunological effect of bromelain and trypsin on mononuclear cells from humans. *European Journal of Medical Research*, volume 10, 325-331.

320. Huang J, et al. (2008). Bromelain inhibits lipopolysaccharide-induced cytokine production in human THP-1 monocytes via the removal of CD14. *Immunological Investigations*, volume 37, 263-277.

321. Fitszhugh D, et al. (2008). Bromelain treatment decreased neutrophil migration to sites of inflammation. *Clinical Immunology*, volume 128, 66-74.

322. Bhui K, et al. (2009). Bromelain inhibits COX-2 expression by blocking the activation of MAPK regulated NF-kappa B against skin tumor-initiation triggering mitochondrial death pathway. *Cancer Letters*, volume 282, 167-176.

323. Kalra N, et al. (2008). Regulation of p53, nuclear factor kappa B and cyclooxygenase-2 expression by bromelain through targeting mitogen-activated protein kinase pathway in mouse skin. *Toxicology and Applied Pharmacology*, volume 226, 30-37.

324. Juhasz B, et al. (2008). Bromelain induces cardioprotection against ischemia-reperfusion injury through Akt/FOXO pathway in rat myocardium. *American Journal of Physiology – Heart and Circulatory Physiology*, volume 294, H1365-H1370.

325. Gerard G. (1972). Therapeutique anti-cancereuse et bromelaine. *Agressologie*, volume 13, 261-274.

326. Nieper H. (1976). Bromelain in der kontrolle malingnen wachstums. *Krebsgeschehen*, volume 1, 9-15.

327. Taussig S, et al. (1985). Inhibition of tumour growth in vitro by bromelain, an extract of the pineapple plant (Ananas comosus). *Planta Medica*, volume 6, 538-539.

328. Garbin F, et al. (1994). Bromelain proteinase F9 augments human lymphocyte-mediated growth and inhibition of various tumor cells in vitro. *International Journal of Oncology*, volume 5, 197-203.

329. Guinmareaes-Ferreira C, et al. (2007). Antitumor effects in vitro and in vivo and mechanisms of protection against melanoma B16F10-Nex2 cells by fastuosain, a cystein proteinase from Bromelia fastuosa. *Neoplasia*, volume 9, 723-733.

330. Tysnes B, et al. (2001). Bromelain reversibly inhibits invasive properties of glioma cells. *Neoplasia*, volume 3, 469-479.

331. Taguchi O, et al. (1997). Prognostic significance of plasma D-dimer levels in patients with lung cancer. *Thorax*, volume 52, 563-565.

332. Dirix L, et al. (2002). Plasma fibrin D-dimer levels correlate with tumour volume, progression and survival in patients with metastatic breast cancer. *British Journal of Cancer*, volume 86, 389-395.

333. Ay C, et al. (2012). High D-dimer levels are associated with poor prognosis in cancer patients. *Haematologica*, volume 97, 1158-1164.

334. Lipinksi B, Egyud L. (2000). Resistance of cancer cells to immune recognition and killing. *Medical Hypotheses*, volume 54, 456-460.

335. Biggerstaff J, et al. (2008). Soluble fibrin inhibits lymphocyte adherence and cytotoxicity against tumor cells: implications for cancer metastasis and immunotherapy. *Clinical and Applied Thrombosis/Hemostasis*, volume 14, 193-202.

336. De-Giuli M, Pirotta F. (1978). Bromelain: interaction with some protease inhibitors and rabbit specific antiserum. *Drugs Under Clinical & Experimental Research*, volume 4, 21-23.

337. Felton G, et al. (1980). Fibrinolytic and antithrombotic action of bromelain may eliminate thrombosis in heart patients. *Medical Hypotheses*, volume 6, 1123-1133.

338. Metzig C, et al. (1999). Bromelain proteases reduce human platelet aggregation in vitro, adhesion to bovine endothelial cells and thrombus formation in rat vessels in vivo. *In Vivo*, volume 13, 7-12.

339. Grignani G, et al. (1989). Mechanisms of platelet activation by cultured human cancer cells and cells freshly isolated from tumor tissues. *Invasion Metastasis*, volume 9, 298-309.

340. McNicol A, Israels S. (2008). Beyond hemostasis: the role of platelets in inflammation, malignancy and infection. *Cardiovascular & Hematological Disorders – Drug Targets*, volume 8, 99-117.

341. Heinicke R, et al. (1972). Effect of bromelain (Ananase®) on human platelet aggregation. *Experientia*, volume 28, 844-845.

342. Morita A, et al. (1979). Chromatographic fractionation and characterization of the active platelet aggregation inhibitory factor from bromelain. *Archives Internationales de Pharmacodynamie et de Therapie*, volume 239, 340-350.

343. Glaser D, Hilberg T. (2006). The influence of bromelain on platelet count and platelet activity in vitro. *Platelets*, volume 17, 37-41.

344. Ley C, et al. (2011). A review of the use of bromelain in cardiovascular diseases. *Journal of Chinese Integrative Medicine*, volume 9, 702-709.

345. Thorne Research (2010). Bromelain monograph. *Alternative Medicine Review*, volume 15, 361-368.

346. Ozcan M, Juhaimi F. (2011). Nutritive value and chemical composition of prickly pear seeds (Opuntia ficus indica L.) growing in Turkey. *International Journal of Food Sciences and Nutrition*, volume 62, 533-536.

347. Rodriguez-Fragoso L, et al. (2008). Risks and benefits of commonly used herbal medicines in Mexico. *Toxicology and Applied Pharmacology*, volume 227, 125-135.

348. Panico A, et al. (2005). Protective effects of Capparis spinosa on chondrocytes. *Life Science*, volume 77, 2479-2488.

349. Zhong X, et al. (2010). Chemical analysis and antioxidant activities in vitro of polysaccharide extracted from Opuntia ficus indica Mill. cultivated in China. *Carbohydrate Polymers*, volume 82, 722-727.

350. Tesoriere L, et al. (2004). Supplementation with cactus pear (Opuntia ficus-indica) fruit decreases oxidative stress in healthy humans: a comparative study with vitamin C. *American Journal of Clinical Nutrition*, volume 80, 391-395.

351. "Whole Grains and Fiber." *Whole Grains and Fiber*. American Heart Association, n.d. Web. 31 Dec. 2012. <http://www.heart.org/HEARTORG/GettingHealthy/NutritionCenter/HealthyDietGoals/Whole-Grains-and-Fiber_UCM_303249_Article.jsp>.

352. Bensadon S, et al. (2010). By-products of Opuntia ficus-indica as a source of antioxidant dietary fiber. *Plant Foods for Human Nutrition*, volume 65, 210-216.

353. Chavez-Santoscoy R, et al (2009). Phenolic composition, antioxidant capacity and in vitro cancer cell cytotoxicity of nine prickly pear (Opuntia spp.) juices. *Plant Foods for Human Nutrition*, volume 64, 146-152.

354. Sreekanth D, et al. (2007). Betanin a betacyanin pigment purified from fruits of Opuntia ficus-indica induces apoptosis in human chronic myeloid leukemia cell line K562. *Phytomedicine*, volume 14, 739-746.

355. Shapiro K, Gong W. (2002). Natural products used for diabetes. *Journal of the American Pharmaceutical Association*, volume 42, 217-226.

356. Roman-Ramos R, et al. (1995). Antihyperglycemic effect of some edible plants. *Journal of Ethnopharmacology*, volume 48, 25-32.

357. Rayburn K, et al. (1998). Glycemic effects of various species of nopal (Opuntia sp.) in type 2 diabetes mellitus. *Texas Journal of Rural Health*, volume 26, 68-76.